The Birth of Penicillin

by the same author

Pomp and Pestilence
An Outline of Bacteriology and Immunity
Bacteriology and Immunity for Nurses
Chapter in Diseases in Antiquity

The Birth of Penicillin

AND THE DISARMING OF MICROBES

RONALD HARE

ILLUSTRATED

London
GEORGE ALLEN AND UNWIN LTD

FIRST PUBLISHED IN 1970

SBN 04 925005 1

The superior numbers in the text are references to sources on page 228

PRINTED IN GREAT BRITAIN
in 11 on 12 Times
BY ALDEN & MOWBRAY LTD
OXFORD

To Barbara
who helped so much

ACKNOWLEDGEMENTS

The author is greatly indebted to the many friends and colleagues who have helped him in the writing of this book, but he must particularly mention Dr W. D. Foster without whose encouragement it is doubtful whether it would have been finished and who was good enough to read the manuscript. He is also grateful to Dr Stuart Craddock, Mr Frederick Ridley, Prof. Reginald Lovell, Dr Albert Fuller and Dr C. J. La Touche who have made available a great deal of information. Amongst others who have helped are Prof. D. M. Pryce, Prof. L. P. Garrod, Dr C. G. Paine, Dr V. D. Allison, Dr K. B. Rogers, Dr L. B. Holt, Dr Howard Hughes, Dr K. P. Hare, Dr Fraser Williams, Dr J. K. W. Ferguson, Dr Mark Ridley, and Mr P. Flood.

He must also record his indebtedness to Miss Madelein Conn for translations and help with the manuscript, Dr Jan Stern for assistance with translations and Mrs Eileen Hardy for secretarial assistance.

Photographic assistance has also been provided by Mr N. G. Le Page, Mr R. Legg, Mr Clifford Smith, and Mr G. D. Wasley for which the author is very grateful.

Thanks are also due to the following: the Director of Her Majesty's Stationery Office, for permission to use data for Figs. 1 and 2, the Association of the British Pharmaceutical Industry for the information on which Fig. 3 is based, the Council of the Wright–Fleming Institute, Bildarchiv J. F. Lehmanns Verlag Munich, and the Photographic Department of St Mary's Hospital Medical School for permission to reproduce photographs, the Managers of the *British Journal of Experimental Pathology* for allowing reproduction of a photograph and quotations and the Editor of *The Practitioner* for quotations.

CONTENTS

ILLUSTRATIONS

PLATES

ILLUSTRATIONS

FIGURES

Chapter 1

Optimism and Bottles of Medicine

Almost everyone now knows that it is possible to prevent some of the diseases caused by microbes such as diphtheria, poliomyelitis and whooping cough by the administration of vaccines but that the great majority cannot be prevented so easily. All that can be done is to treat the patients when they catch the disease. This too is now possible, as a result of this we are rapidly becoming masters of our microbes so that we become infected less often, recover more quickly if we do, and death from an uncomplicated infection is becoming increasingly unusual.

It took about 150 years of trial and experimentation before this was achieved. That infection could be prevented by simple and harmless procedures was first shown to be possible in the closing years of the eighteenth century, when Edward Jenner prevented smallpox by vaccination. The successful treatment of microbial disease had to wait another hundred years. But on Christmas Eve, 1891, a Berlin physician administered antitoxin to a child with diphtheria. She recovered, though but for the antitoxin would have died. Since then so many chemical compounds, sera and antibiotics, have been discovered that very few of the diseases caused by microbes cannot be successfully treated.

It is with this revolution in medicine that this book is mainly concerned. But it is not meant to be a complete history of its inception and development. It is no more than what a fortunately placed observer saw of its progress. For, being born into a medical family in the last August of the nineteenth century and therefore soon after the start of this revolution, never being without close contact with medical practice during my school-days, and eventually making bacteriology my life's work, I was not only a witness but a participant in some of the major events in medical discovery. It is largely because of such close contact that this book has been written.

At the time of my entry into the world my father was the general practitioner in a pit village called Esh Winning, a few miles west of Durham city. It was tacitly assumed from the beginning that when I grew up I would become a doctor, and partly because of this and partly because my mother played an unusually active part in the conduct of the practice, there were few inhibitions in the household about the medical affairs of the village. The impressions I gained as a child were largely confirmed and greatly extended, by my acting, soon after I qualified in 1924, as an assistant in an almost identical practice in a neighbouring valley. In this way I acquired a clear idea of what could be done to prevent and cure disease in a comparatively remote village during the first two decades of this century.

Despite the so-called sanitary reforms of the latter half of the nineteenth century and the passage of the Public Health Act in 1875 that was supposed to bring health and happiness to everyone, very little was actually being done to prevent disease. There may have been a County or even a Rural Medical Officer of Health but their impact on the village cannot have amounted to much. The nearest health officer who was really doing something was probably the Port Medical Officer in Newcastle whose principal activity was the boarding of all incoming vessels to find out how many cases of cholera, plague or smallpox they had on board. It must have been a red-letter day when he found one and he probably spent most of his life in a state of acute boredom.

The procedures we now associate with public health and hygiene may have been mooted at that time, but very few of them were in operation in a small colliery village such as Esh Winning. There were no antenatal or child welfare clinics, no one inspected school children to find out if they had anything wrong with them, there was no control over housing, and very little over water supply or the removal of sewage. So much so that few of the houses had bathrooms, and the colliers who inhabited them had to get themselves clean, when they returned home covered in coal dust, by bathing in a tin bath in front of the kitchen fire. The disposal of the waste products of their metabolism was equally primitive for it amounted to nothing more than a privy in the garden. These were emptied only infrequently, if at all, so that they smelled abominably and, in hot weather, bred flies in such numbers that summer diarrhoea, as gastro-enteritis was frequently called, was not only a common disease but carried off an appreciable number of the younger children. None of the milk was pasteurized but most of it contained tubercle bacilli so that there was a constant succession of children with scrofula, a chronic infection of the glands in the neck; or, what was worse, tuberculosis of the knee, hip or spine with severe crippling if the child was fortunate enough to recover at all.

Even if my father had tried to prevent disease by measures that a general practitioner could initiate, there was very little he could have done. Vitamins had not been invented, so that although rickets was still a common disease he could not suggest its prevention by a more suitable diet than the bread, jam and tea on which so many of the children were brought up. Nor was the connection between diet and caries of the teeth suspected, and quite a number of children reached adult life with few or none to their credit. In fact, the one preventive measure he could employ was to vaccinate against smallpox. But even this was probably less efficient than it was supposed to be; especially in the summer. For the calf lymph required was sent once a month in wooden cylinders about the size of a pencil that my mother subsequently made into needle cases. The package spent most of the time, unopened, on my father's desk where the sun must have cooked the virus within so thoroughly that it is improbable that vaccinations towards the end of the month were as effective as those at the beginning.

Prevention of disease being denied him, most of his energies were devoted to its treatment after it had developed. For this purpose he had, to a large extent, to depend on himself. There was, it is true, an assistant, usually young and only recently qualified who was probably more a liability than an asset. There was also a district nurse, a charming woman who used to take my brother and me out into the woods for picnics. But there was no midwife. I forget the reason but there was, certainly, a profound dislike of them by general practitioners at that time; I suppose they were looked upon as intruders into medical territory. But it meant that many of my father's nights were spent at confinements with only a handywoman for assistance.

Many more of the patients were suffering from the attentions of microbes or viruses than would be the case nowadays, so that their combating was one of his principal occupations. Even so, there was precious little he could do for his patients.

Diphtheria was, and indeed remained for the next 10 years, the only microbial disease for which my father could do anything that was likely to cure it. He gave the patients antitoxin, but so infectious was it considered to be that it was dreaded by everyone, and an important part of the treatment was the prevention of further cases by the removal of the patient in a horsedrawn tumbril of singularly funereal aspect to a fever hospital buried in the depths of the country far from human habitations. Nothing whatever was available for the treatment of scarlet fever which, at that time, was an extremely vicious infection with a high death rate. But it was considered to be equally if not more infectious than diphtheria so that its victims were disposed of in the same way. It is perhaps not surprising that we children were sternly warned to keep as far as possible from the tumbril whenever it appeared in the streets.

In many ways, patients with diseases thought to be so infectious that they had to be put away out of sight and hearing to save the rest of the community, were fortunate because they were, at least, looked after properly. So too were patients with the more dramatic forms of infection such as appendicitis or peritonitis that required operation, because they went to nursing homes or the Royal Infirmaries in Durham or Newcastle. From there, provided they survived the vomiting inseparable from the anaesthesia of those days, they might emerge alive. But for nearly everyone else in the village the only alternative was the poor law infirmary, generally considered to be a place in which to die rather than recover. Because of this, most of them preferred to stay at home and risk it.

The fact remains, however, that at that time microbial diseases were not only commoner but much more severe than they are now. This particularly applied to acute pneumonia and meningitis in their various forms, infections of the urinary and biliary tracts, acute tonsillitis and its sequelae such as otitis media, mastoiditis, quinsy and inflammation of the lymph glands in the neck. Childhood diseases too, abounded, such as acute gastro-enteritis, or cholera infantum as it used to be called; rheumatic fever; chorea and the severe and often fatal complications of measles. If this were not enough, there were the suppurative conditions common at all ages: that is to say, boils, carbuncles, deep abscesses and cellulitis.

Many patients with such conditions would nowadays be sent almost automatically to hospitals, but my father generally had to do the best he could for them at home. He even had to look after patients with pulmonary tuberculosis, only a few being sent to sanatoria. But they were easier to deal with than most because they were generally afflicted with what was called *spes phthisica*, an unfounded optimism that if the cough would only go, as coughs generally do, they would recover. It never did, and they remained at home, cheerfully hoping for recovery almost until the day they died. Typhoid fever, too, was frequently treated at home. The patient was usually left alone, but his immersion in cold water was, at that time, being advocated in the medical schools as the best form of therapy. In the absence of my father, an assistant who tried it was nearly lynched and the treatment was discontinued. The colliers were wiser than the professors.

Being unable to combat microbes by methods likely to kill them, my father was forced to treat patients with infections by the same methods he used for the treatment of other diseases. This was a strange mixture of optimism and bottles of medicine. The optimism, that is to say, making the patient and his family think that everything possible was being done for him, was administered by a process whose basic principle was that it was the doctor who visited the patient, no matter how trivial his illness; the exact opposite of present day practice. Nor was the visit itself conducted in the furtive and surreptitious manner of a debt collector. It was, in its way, an impressive performance involving great attention to transport, dress and deportment.

It started after his morning surgery was over when, immaculately dressed with high linen collar, white cravat and, most important of all, a brown bowler hat, he ascended to the driver's seat of the brightly polished trap in which he did his rounds. I often accompanied him. Whenever we encountered a patient the brown bowler was raised with great dignity, the recipient of the greeting touched his hat – since they were nearly all miners, it was generally a cap – and, the bowler being replaced, we proceeded on our way. Because nearly everyone in the village was or had been a patient, the hat was in an up-and-down motion most of the time. This, aided by the equine propellant of the vehicle, generally gave the whole business something of the *éclat* of a royal procession.

Arrived at the home of a patient, it was only seldom that anything resembling a clinical examination was carried out. In any event, my father's only equipment for the purpose was a stethoscope and his five senses. All he could do was enquire about the patient's progress, suggest something about his diet, say a few words of encouragement, and instruct the family to collect a bottle of medicine at his house that evening. Having produced an aura of totally unfounded optimism in this way, we would then take our seats in the trap and proceed down the street to the next case.

The bottle of medicine was my mother's responsibility. Only four medicaments were available and their compounding could not have been simpler. Three were in liquid form and concentrated solutions of their ingredients were kept ready in the dispensary. When therefore the note my father had written at the bedside telling her what to give was handed in, all she had to do was to add a small quantity to the appropriate amount of water, put the mixture into a bottle, attach a label and give it to the messenger. The whole business would take only a minute or so instead of the hour or more required to extract a comparable mixture from a chemist nowadays.

By far the most popular of these mixtures was *Mist tussis*, in other words, a cough mixture. Compounded of bromide of ammonia and belladaonna, flavoured with camphor, it was given for practically every disease of the respiratory tract, whether or not it was caused by microbes. When the symptoms were below the diaphragm, two mixtures were available. The first, containing bicarbonate of soda and extract of rhubarb, was accordingly known as *Mist soda cum rhei.* Its taste was foul and its odour objectionable but it was a sovereign remedy for acute upsets of the digestive tract. The cure was almost worse than the disease. For less acute conditions, *Mist alba* was equally valuable. It was also kinder to both the olfactory and gustatory senses because it consisted of peppermint water containing Epsom salt and magnesium carbonate. The fourth remedy at my mother's disposal was a package of six teething powders. They were given freely and often, because practically every form of illness in young children was considered to be connected with the eruption of teeth. As these powders contained mercury and chalk, mild mercurial poisoning was almost an occupational hazard of infancy at that time.

Their preparation was a more complicated business than that of the bottled mixtures. It generally took place in the evenings on the dining-room table. I frequently assisted in the process but it required long practice to acquire the skill necessary to fold the squares of paper in which they were packed so that the powder would remain within them. But I was not allowed, for obvious reasons, to apply the blob of sealing wax that secured the outer wrapper in which six of the powders were enclosed.

My father died soon after I had become proficient in the art of packaging powders but I still maintained contact with medicine, because many school holidays were spent with uncles who were general practitioners. The methods they used were almost exactly the same as my father's. Even an uncle who lived in rural Hertfordshire and prided himself on his keeping up with progress by regular attendance at the meetings of the Cambridge Medical Society, could not improve on them.

Nevertheless, it was during this period that there came the first real advance since the introduction of diphtheria antitoxin in 1891. This was the synthesis of a compound containing arsenic that could cure syphilis. I was only ten years old at the time, too young to be told about it. But, with this exception, the active treatment of microbial infections cannot be said to have progressed very far during my schooldays.

In 1919, having won the scholarship that was essential if I was to achieve my ambition, I became a medical student at St Mary's Hospital in London. It was probably because it was, at that time, one of the least distinguished of the medical schools that they accepted me. In fact, although I did not know it at the time, the school had only recently been condemned by the University Grants Committee as being unsuitable for its purpose. It was only rescued from closure by its dean, Dr Charles Wilson, better known as Lord Moran.

It is not surprising that the committee had been so pessimistic about its future because it would be difficult to imagine a more unprepossessing an institution. Even its environment was unfortunate. In the South Wharf Road near Paddington station, whose farther side was flanked by a series of warehouses backing on to the Grand Union Canal, it was chiefly used by the Great Western Railway vans on their way to and from Paddington Goods Station. Their iron-shod wheels rattled over the cobblestones to such good purpose that many of the patients in the nearby wards were wakened much too early. The horses, too, were stabled next door to the medical school, so that if one could not hear them one could frequently smell them.

Entered by a mean doorway from this thoroughfare, the school itself was an equally mean three-storied building of red brick that had acquired a rich patina of grime. Its interior was little better. The corridors were of stone, and because it depended on coal fires, most of which were never lit, it was cold and draughty in the winter. There was a singularly uninviting staircase that ended at the dissecting room, a white-tiled barn of a place with windows and skylight so obscured by grime that the pathetic objects on the table looked even more repulsive than they need have done. But the height of discomfort was reached in its main lecture theatre. This consisted of a series of semicircles of hard wooden benches with very slender back rests fronted by another series of semicircles about 6 inches wide, supported on infrequent iron rods that were supposed to do duty as desks. Its one merit was that the seats were so uncomfortable that it was impossible to do anything but listen to the lecture. Sleep, illicit reading of newspapers or even doodling were all out of the question.

In view of all this, it is not surprising that the school possessed too many deficiencies to be of much value as a centre of learning and research. Even a medical student could see that there was nowhere to do it, very little technical help and virtually no apparatus. Much of this was due to the fact that, although recognized by the University of London as one of its schools, St Mary's was, like most of the other schools, completely independent and owned by the parent hospital. If it received money from the hospital it cannot have amounted to much because the latter still largely depended on voluntary contributions. So poor was it that when Almroth Wright became pathologist in the early years of the century and desired to to do research in the evenings, he was seriously impeded by the fact that the hospital authorities cut off the electric supply to his laboratory at 6.00 p.m., the theory being, no doubt, that no useful pathology was likely to be done at a time when ordinary individuals were on their way home to dress for dinner. Wright, who seldom ate before 9.00 p.m. and never dressed for it unless he had to, found the lack of illumination a serious impediment. But the authorities had omitted to turn off the gas so that John Freeman, one of his assistants, was able to come to the rescue by placing incandescent mantles on two bunsen burners, and Wright was able to pursue his researches untrammelled by darkness. I have reason to believe that some other institutions of higher learning were equally parsimonious at that time.

To do them credit, however, our teachers did at least instruct us sufficiently in the rudiments of anatomy, physiology and biochemistry to enable me to pass the necessary examinations in the spring of 1921, and I then started to walk the wards. Here the environment was slightly better. Hospitals are usually kept clean. But intellectually, it was much the same. Except possibly for the fact that the surgeons did operations that frequently cured the patients, the treatment of other diseases was almost exactly the same as that which my father had given his patients in the pit village in Durham. Like all students of those days I first came into contact with them in the casualty department. Here, in addition to the setting of fractures and the extraction of teeth, we learned to stitch wounds, and in the hope of preventing the otherwise inevitable suppuration anointed them with antiseptics. Not the tincture of iodine my father had used, but a paste known as B.I.P.P. said to have been invented by a President of the Royal College of Surgeons and, because of this, considered to be an unfailing prophylactic. It was not, but it did possess a penetrating odour of iodoform. The patient was, accordingly, liable to be asked awkward questions when he got home because some of the family probably knew that this compound was also used for the treatment of gonorrhoea.

If he had acquired this disease he was dealt with less publicly, in a remote corner of the hospital. All that could be done for him were frequent and extremely painful irrigations with an antiseptic solution of some kind. The treatment of syphilis was even more rigorous for it necessitated about thirty weekly injections of the arsenical preparation to which I have already referred. But all this did at least cure the disease, which is more than could be said for most methods of treatment at that time.

For the treatment of local infections such as boils, nothing even remotely resembling penicillin was available. Here too we used fundamentally the same treatment as my father's. We brought the boils to a head with hot fomentations and lanced them, but with the added refinement that the patient was anaesthetized; or, more correctly, was partially asphyxiated by gas and struggling violently. This meant that the operation had to be conducted in a great hurry. I have often wondered why we so seldom cut ourselves in the process and infected ourselves in turn.

After three months of this I became intimately acquainted with deeper and more serious forms of infection in the wards. They were full of patients with acute pneumonia, empyema, typhoid fever, infected compound fractures and burns, many forms of tuberculosis, syphilitic lesions such as gummata and locomotor ataxia, uncontrollable infections of the bones called osteomyelitis, rheumatic fever and its irreparable injuries to the heart, and even rare diseases like tetanus. We also attended fever hospitals where we saw diphtheria cases by the hundred, not to mention scarlet fever, measles and mumps. But wherever we went, the treatment was much the same as that given by my father in the remote village in Durham.

In all this, St Mary's was no better and no worse than other hospitals of the period. Some of the clinicians may have realized that, as they were the leaders of the profession, they should be doing something more towards finding ways and means of treating their patients more satisfactorily. But most of them spent only two half-days a week at it. The rest of their time was spent on private patients, who were their sole source of income. The hospital paid them nothing whatever for their services. They accordingly spent a great deal of their time travelling to see the patients who were scattered all over London in their own homes or in the many nursing homes that existed at that time. Some had difficulty in finding time to eat. Sir William Broadbent, one of the foremost heart specialists at the turn of the century, often had to have recourse to a rice pudding his cook had thoughtfully concealed in the recesses of his brougham before he left in the morning.

Small wonder that few of them made the slightest attempt to do any form of research. They would have had to see fewer patients or give up their leisure. Even so, there was nowhere to do it. The only laboratory at St Mary's to which they had access was a tiny room in the basement where the medical clerks tested urine. Prof. Langmead had one which was larger because he was professor of medicine, but this was a very recent innovation, and in any event, its one technician and all its resources were occupied in the manufacture of insulin, not yet commercially available. The laboratory occupied by Dr Roche Lynch was also out of bounds. Although it carried out some of the more elaborate biochemical tests needed by the patients, its main activity was the detection of poisons in the bodies of victims of murder.

For the treatment of their patients, their resources were little better than those of my father. The clinicians were, it is true, better dressed and their transport was more luxurious. But their psychological effect on their hospital patients at least, was very much worse. Indeed, on the days they visited their wards the latter had been in a furore since early morning preparing for the arrival of the great man, with Sister not far short of hysteria and the nurses dead beat with fatigue by the time he arrived. The prevailing apprehension had communicated itself to the patients who were now tucked up so securely in bed that they could hardly move. Not that they were encouraged to do so; it might have disturbed the symmetry of the spotlessly clean sheets and counterpanes in which they were encased. And woe betide the unfortunate patient whose metabolism had become so deranged that he had to have a bed pan about the time the great man arrived. Small wonder that most of them were speechless with fear when the door opened and he swept into his realm.

Not that he did much when he finally reached them. The optimism my father had generated was conspicuous by its absence. In fact, the patient was fortunate if the consultant went so far as to look at him and even more so if there was any indication that the object in the bed was a human being.

The little optimism that was meted out came from the Sisters in charge of the wards. Even so, it cannot have amounted to much because they were all starched to the eyebrows and so formidable of aspect that any words of encouragement they may have uttered would have been largely neutralized by their appearance. Bottles of medicine were, of course, provided. The prescriptions may have been more elegant and contained more ingredients, but they were no more efficient than those my mother had dispensed years before.

I qualified in the summer of 1924 by passing the examinations of the Society of Apothecaries which, considering my subsequent career, could not have been more appropriate. Had I attended any of the other London hospitals, I would probably have become insusceptible to the prevailing impotence in the face of so much disease, and taken up some form of clinical medicine. Even if I had made an attempt to dissipate some of the impotence, I would probably have had to give up the struggle for no other reason than sheer lack of opportunities. But, unlike all the other London schools, St Mary's possessed one of the foremost bacteriological research laboratories in the country at that time. Housed in converted wards fronting on to Praed Street, it was known as the Inoculation Department. Despite its utilitarian nomenclature it had already gained a formidable reputation for its work on the prevention and treatment of bacterial diseases.

Although as students we had seldom penetrated so far, I had seen it when we were on the way to receive instruction in bacteriology. I do not think I will ever forget my first sight of the upstairs laboratory, into which we could see through large glass doors on the way to the lecture room. There were white-tiled benches at which sat four men entirely concentrated on what they were doing. The room itself was in semi-darkness but their benches were brightly illuminated by shaded lamps. There was a bright fire burning at one end, there seemed to be an abundance of apparatus about, much of it of brass and all highly polished. The place had an air of real purpose about it.

The practical classes were conducted with an efficiency unknown in the medical school. There were not only several technicians to fetch and carry but some of the men I had just seen in the laboratory emerged to act as demonstrators. What is more, each student's place was properly prepared for him with rows of stains all ready, blotting paper, slides and cultures.

How very different all this was from what I had seen in the medical school. Few of the teachers ever did any research at all. They had probably given up the struggle long ago. There was generally only one technician to look after a whole department, the laboratories were stone cold most of the winter, they were thick with dust and there was very little apparatus, a great deal of it broken or out of action.

This was the first time I had seen a properly run laboratory in which a real attempt was being made to do research. And, moreover, by men who, when viewed from the back in dim light, seemed utterly devoted to their work.

Is it then so very surprising that having seen, ever since my childhood, how ineffective was the treatment of illness and how little was being done in the medical schools to put matters right, I began to feel rebellious? And so, quite early in my student days, I determined that, if it would have me, I would get a job in the only place I knew where some progress was being made.

Chapter 2

Antibodies, Antiseptics and Arsenic

At the time I qualified, anyone wanting to do medical research usually started by getting a job in the pathology department of a teaching hospital. Like his chief, his principal activity would have been the performance of post-mortem examinations and the microscopic study of specimens removed at operations to ascertain whether the patient had cancer. And largely because both of them knew how to look down a microscope, they would have done the rudimentary haematology and bacteriology of those days. They might even have ventured into biochemical territory, but this would have been unusual because its exploration was only seldom required.

Despite these preoccupations, the young man might have succeeded in doing some research. But having given up his spare time for a year or so in order to do it, he had probably found that the game was not worth the candle. He would continue with his routine investigations until, after endless lobbyings and schemings, he would obtain an appointment as pathologist in some hospital where he eked out his inadequate salary by performing post-mortem examinations for coroners and pathological investigations for the private patients of the specialists.

Although I might have had a more peaceful and even more prosperous life if I had followed this course, the existence of the Inoculation Department barred all further progress in that direction. For it not only encouraged research but paid thirteen or fourteen men to do it.

What is more, it gave scholarships of £200 a year to young

men wanting to do research; and, one becoming available soon after I had taken my London degree, I applied and was accepted. And so, without benefit of even an internship and still less a postgraduate qualification, but far, far more important, when only 25 years old and still possessing the youthful enthusiasm the modern system of training so effectively dissipates before a man starts his life's work, I entered the laboratory that was to be my scientific home for the next 6 years.

I do not propose to say very much about the previous history of the Department. It has been quite adequately described in the biographies of Wright[10] and Fleming[63] Suffice it to say that it made bacteriological history early in the century by introducing a method of treatment for bacterial infections known as vaccine therapy, the best description of which may be found, strange to say, in the first act of George Bernard Shaw's play, *The Doctor's Dilemma*. When the First World War broke out, most of the staff became officers in the R.A.M.C. and migrated to Boulogne, where they carried out research on wound infections that had a profound effect on the methods of treatment employed during and after the war. When they returned to St Mary's after the armistice, their activities became more diverse. Attempts were, for example, made to treat severe infections by an unusual form of blood transfusion; Fleming discovered lysozyme, an important natural protective substance, and studied it intensively with Dr V. D. Allison for several years; and John Freeman became an authority on the causation and relief of asthma and hay fever, the introduction of pollen extract for the prevention of the latter being one of his achievements.

All this was to its credit at the time I started to work in the Department, but in 1928 came its most outstanding achievement, the discovery of penicillin. Thus, quite by chance, within a month or two of my qualification, I found myself in a laboratory that had already made a name for itself and was soon to become even better known.

Nevertheless, for all its distinction, it was very unlike the research laboratories of the present day with their palatial entrances, air-conditioned offices, wide corridors and abundance of secretaries and technicians. So much so, that I may be forgiven if I describe it in a little more detail if only to emphasize the fact that it is not bricks and mortar that make discoveries but the brains that they shelter. For many years, the Department consisted of laboratories adapted from four wards originally designed to hold six or seven patients on the first and second floors of St Mary's at its south-east corner facing on to Praed Street. In 1933 it migrated to a splendid new building on the other side of Norfolk Place, and in 1945 its utilitarian nomenclature gave way to the Wright–Fleming Institute of Microbiology. But the laboratories in which I worked and in which penicillin was discovered were very different. They were, for example, hopelessly overcrowded. No one, not even Wright, its Director, had a private office and all of us did our work and even our writing on about 6 feet of bench, in rooms some of which were inhabited by as many as six other people. Privacy was completely unknown. The commercial activities of the place, on which its finances depended, were compressed into two rooms not more than about 15 feet square. The room in which all the glassware was prepared and the media made was not very much larger. The darkroom had been converted from a very small w.c. and the hot room was a gas-operated deathtrap about the same size.

Although the Department had appeared much more prosperous and better staffed than any I had seen in the Medical School as a student, it was almost poverty-stricken by modern standards. We had to buy our own microscopes. There was no fume cupboard or sterile room. The nearest approach to a refrigerator was a wooden box about the size of a tea chest into which someone inserted a block of ice if he happened to remember. But one thing the place did possess, and in abundance, was its smell: an all-pervading odour of hot oil reminiscent of an engine room, which was produced by the heated oil baths in which we sterilized our syringes.

Poverty-stricken, ill-equipped and smelly though it may have been, it was never, like the laboratories in the medical school, dirty and untidy. All the brassware, most of the apparatus was made of it, shone brightly; the white-tiled benches were cleaned every morning and there was always a cheerful fire in the winter.

Technicians were few and far between; each man was expected to do all his own work. Personal secretaries were unknown. Letters were generally written in longhand and scientific papers picked out with forefingers on the portable typewriters most of us possessed. Photography had to be done by the man who required it and he would have had to use his own camera. The preparation of lantern slides required such superhuman ingenuity that it was generally avoided. Lectures were illustrated by placards that might measure 4 feet square.

For all its physical limitations it was, in fact, a comparatively wealthy institution. It was certainly the most prosperous part of St Mary's. Since 1908, when it was founded, it had made vaccines in quantity for sale to practitioners through a firm of pharmaceutical chemists. This enabled it to do something almost unique at that time, pay salaries to young men who wanted to do research. Minute salaries it is true, but just sufficient to enable a bachelor to live. In any event, some of them supplemented them with fees from private practice. Most of the older men in the place, when I started to work in it, had been recruited in this way.

From 1908 until 1945 its Chief was Sir Almroth Wright, one of the most remarkable men who ever entered medicine. Full details of his life may be found in the biographies by Colebrook[10] and by Cope,[15] while I myself have written an appraisal of his scientific work.[48] As he wielded immense influence over the men in his own department as well as in the world outside, it is necessary that I say something about him.

His first real opportunity had come when he was appointed Professor of Pathology in 1892, at the age of 31, at the Royal Army Medical College, at that time part of the Royal Victoria Hospital at Netley on the banks of Southampton Water. Here he soon made bacteriological history by inventing a vaccine for the prevention of typhoid fever which is, in all essentials, the same as that used today. In 1902 he was appointed pathologist at St Mary's Hospital but resigned in 1908 to become Director of the Inoculation Department. Until the outbreak of the First World War he developed and employed a method of treatment known as vaccine therapy. But in 1914 he and most of his staff migrated to Boulogne where, in a makeshift laboratory in the fencing school on the roof of the Casino, they studied infection of wounds until the end of the War. He then returned to St Mary's, retired in 1945, and died in 1947.

In his prime, that is to say, from the turn of the century until the end of the First World War, he had been a well-known public figure largely because he could never behave in the same way as other people. Indeed, his own mother complained that he was the only member of her numerous family who never did as he was told.

It is not, therefore, surprising that he became a medical nuisance of the first order. He never missed an opportunity of pillorying Harley Street for its old-fashioned methods of medical practice, getting himself dubbed the Prophet from Praed Street by one of the medical journals for his pains. And towards the end of the First World War he succeeded in making himself thoroughly detested by most of the medical profession for publishing what can only be described as a masterpiece of sustained invective attacking the then President of the Royal College of Surgeons.

It is perhaps not surprising that with such a person in charge his laboratory was ruled with a rod of iron. Every member of the team had to support him and his somewhat revolutionary ideas wholeheartedly. The few that could not do so got out, but amongst those who accepted these conditions were some of the best brains in the profession.

Amongst those who had been his pupils at Netley, for example, were Sir William Leishman, Sir David Semple, Sir Leonard Rogers, Col. S. Lyle Cummins and Col. L. W. Harrison, all of whom have made notable contributions to bacteriology. It was much the same after he came to St Mary's where, in addition to Alexander Fleming, he soon recruited John Freeman, S. R. Douglas, Leonard Colebrook and Leonard Noon. None of them was without some influence on bacteriology or immunity. Because of this it is, perhaps, not surprising that amongst his pupils there was one Nobel Laureate, a Director-General of the R.A.M.C., four Fellows of the Royal Society, a Fellow of the Royal Society of Canada, and several

Directors of research institutes and occupants of university chairs.

A tireless worker himself, he expected his men to work as hard as he did. Those he had recruited in the early days of the depart ment had all worked, for minute salaries, far into the night because the tests they were using to control vaccine therapy could not be started until after dinner in the evening; most of the day was spent in seeing patients and collecting the necessary specimens. In consequence, few of them got home before midnight. Prof. Carmalt Jones once told me that while he was working there one summer, the dawn was usually breaking as he walked home. This nocturnal mode of existence was invariably referred to when post-war recruits such as myself grumbled about staying late, and led to the convention that any research carried out in daylight could not be worth very much.

When the war was over and Wright returned to St Mary's, things became slightly more normal. Most of the team he had ruled with so firm a hand remained with him it is true, but they had grown too old to dance to his tune and were going their own ways. The one-time dictator retreated into his shell, taking very little interest in what the old hands or even new recruits like myself were doing. Indeed, within reason, they all could do as they liked, and it was only when unusual expenditure was required or the draft of a paper was submitted before publication, that he took much interest. But for all its disparate activities the team still held together, largely because the events of the past years had given Wright and his men an extraordinary sense of *élan*. The survivors were a team of friends who had been through fire and water together.

Lest this corporate spirit should die out, they had evolved the custom of taking tea together every day without fail; the ceremony, for it was just that, taking place in the library. Although only about 12 feet square and already encumbered by a desk and divan, it managed to hold regularly no less than twelve and sometimes many more people.

The proceedings were dominated by Wright. All that he required was an audience and someone to talk back at him. This was the main function of Freeman in the place, the rest of us kept quiet, it was the safest thing to do. But it was a first-rate education, for although Wright seems never to have met Pasteur, he knew practically all the other pioneers. Whatever was going on in the laboratories was also discussed, but it must not be concluded that all these discussions concerned science or scientists. The fact that Fry had bought a house was the signal for a long discussion on gardens, that Craddock was about to be married provided another on the foibles of the female sex, and that I painted pictures required the production of one for inspection and a long lecture on colour shadows, the manner of producing which happened to be one of Wright's hobbies.

These daily sessions at the tea-table, some of which lasted as much as an hour, and which went on week after week throughout the year, were not only good training but gave us an insight into the characters of our elders that could have been obtained in no other way.

Wright also became more broad-minded. Even doubts about some of his doctrines were no longer the mortal sins they had once been; so much so that one could even question the validity of some of his techniques without risking expulsion, a fate that would have been almost inevitable before the war. Even more remarkable is the fact that, despite his reputed abomination of chemotherapy, his favourite pupil and closest friend, Colebrook, studied little else for the best part of 20 years.

The erstwhile public figure also disappeared from view. There were no more polemics or letters to the newspapers. There was the occasional flash of the old fire as when, at a meeting of the Royal Society of Medicine, he told Lord Horder who was then at the pinnacle of his fame, that instead of talking about bacterial endocarditis he should do some research on it. But when in 1928 he and George Bernard Shaw took part in a debate on the medical profession and we all expected a display of fireworks, it was no more than a sad spectacle of two old men trying to recapture some of the sparkle that had illuminated similar debates in their younger days.

When, therefore, I first got to know him, he had become, to me at all events, a rather charming old gentleman who had been known for many years as 'The Old Man'. No wonder, for he looked a great deal older than his 64 years, being tall and large of frame with a slightly shambling gait and pronounced stoop. His hair and moustache had become snow white and his eyes were only partially visible behind old-fashioned steel-rimmed spectacles, with bifocal lenses separated by an unusually prominent straight line instead of the invisible curve that is customary. His clothes tended to hang from him rather than fit him, and he invariably wore a stiff wing collar with a tie whose knot was usually anywhere but where it ought to have been.

He seemed quite content to live a well-ordered and peaceful existence, studying a phenomenon known round the place as 'immunity in vitro' when he pottered into the laboratory at 3.00 p.m. until he left for dinner some time after 7.00 p.m. The rest of his waking hours were spent in the composition of a book on logic that was not published until after his death. His only relaxations seemed to be the daily sessions at the tea-table, his garden at Farnham Royal, dinners with the Royal Society Dining Club, and the meetings of the Medical Research Club. He seldom attended the meetings of other scientific societies and avoided membership of committees.

His marriage had broken up before the First World War and he lived in solitary state in a house in Pembroke Square where he was looked after by a housekeeper. But he also had a house at Farnham Royal to which he went every week-end and, when he was 64 years old, actually bought and learned to drive a motor-car to get himself there.

Among the few friends he seemed to have, the Colebrooks were by far the closest; they built a house close to his at Farnham Royal so that he could have company at the week-ends. Dorothy Colebrook kept an eye on his domestic arrangements and Colebrook acted as his amanuensis in the laboratory. He helped him with his lectures, transported him to them and prepared the demonstrations for them. He tried, usually without success, to persuade Wright to stay at home when he got colds or bronchitis, and even made arrangements to get his hair cut. This operation might well have been postponed indefinitely had not Colebrook produced in the laboratory, once a month, a strangely obsequious little man in a state of tremendous excitement over the privilege of cutting the locks of one so distinguished.

Colebrook never lost his devotion for his master. He not only wrote his biography but never missed an opportunity of singing his praises. And woe betide anyone – as I was forced to do on one occasion – who doubted anything done by his hero.

Nevertheless, all through the years, infuriating, argumentative as he could be, obstinate to the point of stupidity, employing experimental methods that were so crude and inaccurate that they almost made one weep, he was, for all this, an inspiration to many generations of younger men, whatever his detractors – and they were many – might say.

Such then was the Department, and its Chief, in which I started work on New Year's day, 1925. My immediate superior was Dr John Freeman, a well known allergist who was also nominally in charge of the routine bacteriological investigations for the hospital. Nominally, I say, because they were all done by Dr C. B. Dyson, who was helped at that time by Dr Ian Maclean, a New Zealander. They were kind enough to take the very raw beginner in hand and in the next month or so I learned a great deal.

Although safely launched in this way, it was not long before I became apprehensive as to whether I could remain afloat. It emerged in the course of conversation that J. F., as Freeman was usually called, was the son of a Mr Freeman who lived in a large house overlooking the river at Halliford Bend, not far from Shepperton. He was a magistrate and, I think, looked upon himself as the squire of the neighbourhood. When, therefore, the erection of about twenty bungalows on a piece of flat marshy land of no particular scenic value, but in full view of his drawing-room windows, was mooted in 1922, he was so horror-stricken that he did everything he could to prevent this unseemly intrusion on his privacy. The attempts had failed and the bungalows were duly erected.

Unfortunately, one of them, which happened to be the most prominent, had been bought by my mother, and with her and my sister I lived in it for the next 5 years. We had little to fear from Freeman *père* while we were in residence because he invariably averted his eyes when propelling the ancient punt in which he occasionally made an evening promenade on the river. But Freeman *fils* occasionally visited his father and did likewise. Being less disturbed about the bungalows, he looked them square in the face. What would have happened had he seen me on one of the verandas I do not like to think, because in those days one's private affairs were less private and heads of departments much less charitable than they are now. Fortunately, he had a very loud voice and no compunction about using it for conversation with the lady passengers he usually took out with him. It was this that, on more than one occasion, saved me and I was able to retire in time. So far as I know, Freeman never learned of the annoyance I had so unwittingly caused his father, because he always thought I lived at Twickenham where I happened to be staying on the one occasion when he asked me where I lived.

Although I always had to keep a weather eye, or perhaps more correctly, ear open when in the front garden, Freeman seldom visited his father. He was too busy with his practice. He also ran two enormous clinics in the laboratory, the patients attending it filling the corridors outside before they were admitted to the tiny cubicle in a corner, in which he gave them injections for asthma and hay fever, his two main interests. In consequence of all this activity he was perpetually in a hurry, and tended to leave me to my own devices. Perhaps this was as well for he was so slapdash on the rare occasions on which he ever did any research that I might have learned bad habits. It was not long, therefore, before I had to branch out on my own and spent most of the year studying the skin reactions in hay fever and similar allergies. As a result, I must have been one of the first to show that histamine plays an important part in producing the symptoms of these diseases. But possibly of greater importance was the fact that, as the work was an outcome of his, I not only got to know Sir Thomas Lewis, one of the great pioneers of clinical research, but learned from him much more about the proper way to do research and describe the experiments than I would ever have learned from Freeman.

Towards the end of the year Leonard Colebrook, who was invariably known as Coli, asked me if I would like to help him when the research scholarship came to an end in December. It transpired that he needed an assitant for his work on puerperal fever, who was to be paid £300 a year by the Medical Research Council. But I was not to assume that this would lead, at any time in the near or distant future, to the permanent appointment with that body which was at that time the standard ambition of anyone aspiring to do medical research. In fact, I was clearly to understand that the salary was dependent on a grant which would be reviewed every year and that it could be terminated whenever Colebrook, the Medical Research Council, the Inoculation Department, or in fact anyone, got tired of me. There was, of course, no pension; no one thought of pensions in 1926. But I was expected to work 24 hours a day and, to facilitate this, was to live as close to St Mary's as possible.

Imagine any young man of the present day accepting a job on those terms, but I agreed to all of them except the last. With a mother to support and a sister to educate, I could not live in London. It was much too expensive. Colebrook had, accordingly, to waive this condition. But it was a blot on my escutcheon. It was not in the true tradition of self-denial required by the Inoculation Department.

Thus began, in this rather casual fashion, not only a lifelong friendship but 10 years association with him which gave me opportunities of witnessing the start of the revolution in medicine that the discovery of penicillin and the sulphonamides brought about. At the beginning of January 1926, as a very temporary, very much on sufferance beginner, I moved into the laboratory upstairs which I had seen from the corridor 6 years before. Here worked Wright and his two assistants, E. J. Storer and R. M. Fry; I. H. Maclean who was studying caries in teeth; A. F. Hayden who did the Wassermans; Colebrook and myself.

At the time I entered the 'House of Lords' as the upstairs laboratory was sometimes called, very little could yet be done to prevent or cure most forms of bacterial and virus infection. And although I have been censorious of the apparent lack of interest on the part of my teachers in the medical school, others, particularly the great pioneers in continental laboratories such as Pasteur, Koch, Ehrlich, Bordet, Metchnikoff and Von Behring, had strained every nerve to find ways and means of curing infected patients. But too little was known about the mechanisms involved in immunity, the sources of the organisms or the ways in which they entered the bodies of their victims, to enable them to achieve very much. It was largely because of this that most microbes flourished in the community without let or hindrance, and if recovery from infection occurred it was usually because nature had willed it so.

Nevertheless, although I did not realize it at the time, these pioneers had either died or had become too old to do very much, and the impetus they had given to research on methods for the cure of disease was dying away. The younger men were not painting such vast canvases. None of them proclaimed, as their scientific fathers had done, that they hoped to save humanity from its microbes. In fact most of them were veering in the opposite direction, and if they were saving anything it seemed to be the microbes they were studying rather than their possible victims; at all events, they were taking more interest in them than in the diseases they caused.

As it happened, however, the Inoculation Department still retained something of the crusading spirit of the bacteriological pioneers. This was almost certainly due to Wright who was, bacteriologically speaking, Victorian rather than Georgian in outlook. He and his men accordingly had no compunction about proclaiming that they were primarily interested in the prevention and cure of disease. If, therefore, I wanted to do something along these lines I had probably chosen the one place in the world that was old-fashioned enough to sympathize with me. But what is of equal importance, it possessed collectively, more experience than any other institution on this subject. In view of what is to follow, it may therefore be appropriate if I describe what the position was, at the time I started to work in it.

Before going into details it is essential to stress that we must distinguish clearly between the prevention of disease and the cure of an infection that has become established, because in general, techniques suitable for the one are different from those required by the other.

Let us therefore consider the prevention of disease first of all. By the mid 1920s, it had become well established that many cases of typhoid, cholera and dysentery could be prevented by the relatively simple process of keeping the microbes away from potential victims by ensuring a pure water supply and the prompt removal of sewage. But the vast majority of infections could not be prevented so easily. A few more could be prevented by making potential victims resistant to infection. This had first been shown to be possible by Edward Jenner when he discovered that vaccination would prevent smallpox. Pasteur, too, had found that rabies need not result if those bitten by rabid dogs were given injections of suspensions made from the spinal cords of rabbits infected by the virus that causes the disease.

The vaccines used for these purposes consisted of living organisms whose virulence had been attenuated in various ways. This made them, theoretically at least, safe. But the founding father of the Inoculation Department had himself made bacteriological history by demonstrating that a living vaccine was not necessary. One consisting of a suspension of killed typhoid bacilli could prevent typhoid fever following its injection. This was a very important step in the history of immunization because there was considerable doubt whether the virulence of some species could be attenuated sufficiently to make them safe enough, and even if this was achieved there was always a risk that for no particular reason they might revert to their original virulent condition.

Nevertheless, even a safe vaccine is usually looked upon with suspicion and Wright was soon to find, as many others have done since, that the evolution of vaccines is child's play compared with the struggles that are required to have them adopted. This was the position that had been reached about the time that Wright left Netley and came to St Mary's. And although neither the hospital nor the Inoculation Department had played any direct part in the evolution of the vaccine, they witnessed at close hand what happened afterwards.

This was a consequence of the fact that, although typhoid was becoming rare in the civilian population, it had almost reached the status of an occupational disease in the army. It was, for example, a common cause of invaliding from India. But it had become a very serious problem during the South African War for it caused more casualties than the enemy's missiles. The War Office had, accordingly, to decide whether or not to use the vaccine. The military medical hierarchy being unable to make up its mind for it, the War Office adopted the usual expedient of any government department when faced with an insoluble problem, and appointed a committee. Not to be outdone, the Royal College of Physicians appointed another. Wright was, of course, on both of them. So, unfortunately, was Sir David Bruce and he combined the advantages of being already a member of the military medical hierarchy and quite as distinguished a bacteriologist as Wright. If this were not enough, he was quite as fiery as Wright and had no use for the vaccine or its inventor. Small wonder that the proceedings of these committees had, as the *British Medical Journal* put it, 'the proverbial mark of true love that did not run smooth'.

Wright did nothing to improve the situation by writing a letter to *The Times* advocating the early adoption of his vaccine. This provoked an almost libellous editorial from the *British Medical Journal* attacking him for using the public press to further his own ends. Nor did the publication by Wright of a little book describing the incidence of the disease in immunized and unimmunized populations help matters.[75] For this roused the wrath of no less a person than Professor Karl Pearson, the eminent mathematician, who wrote a blistering criticism in the *British Medical Journal.* This led to a polemic in the course of which he wrote four more letters, and Wright four in reply. They are well worth reading, even today, for they show what manner of men our forefathers were. In all this Wright was doomed from the start, for he was no match for his opponent on statistical matters, and all he could do was to plead that Pearson had not appreciated the difficulties involved in enquiries of this nature.

All this controversy had one good result. Colonel W. B. Leishman, who had been one of Wright's pupils and eventually became a most distinguished Director-General of the R.A.M.C., was sent to India to carry out what the War Office ought to have done in the beginning, a controlled trial. This vindicated Wright's claims and the vaccine was adopted.

With all this in its archives, it is no exaggeration to say that the Inoculation Department knew more than most research institutes about prophylactic immunization, but in view of what it had gone through in the process it understandably showed little enthusiasm for further excursions into this territory. It accordingly paid little heed to other measures of this nature that had been or were being evolved at the time of which I am speaking. These included the plague and cholera vaccines that Haffkine had developed in India, or those that prevent diphtheria whose value was then being demonstrated in America.[65]

The treatment of infections once they have become established in the tissues is, as I have already mentioned, an entirely different proposition from their prevention. And it was on this aspect of the matter that the Inoculation Department had chiefly concentrated ever since its foundation. For many years, in fact until the sulphonamides appeared, there were three ways in which it was, theoretically at least, possible to treat infections. The first was by immunological methods: that is to say, measures that will assist the natural antibacterial defences of the patient to deal with the invading organisms. The second was by the administration of chemical compounds usually known as antiseptics, that can kill any form of living cell including those of microbes. The third was by another series of chemical compounds collectively known as chemotherapeutic agents that act on the invading organisms but have little effect on the cells of the patient. The Department had played or was about to play a notable part in the study of all three methods.

Although this book is largely concerned with the third of these methods, the use of penicillin being by far the most important, modern chemotherapy might not have been evolved at all if the other methods had been more successful. They did, therefore, play some part, even if it was largely negative, in the development of chemotherapy as we know it today. In order, therefore, to put the matter into its proper perspective, I propose to summarize the position that had been reached by the time that penicillin was discovered.

Immunological methods for the treatment of infections can be defined as techniques in which the mechanisms by which we normally combat microbes are exploited in such a manner as to increase the chance that the patient will recover from the infection. A number of different mechanisms are involved in this process, most of which need not be mentioned, but by far the most important are those that involve the presence of antibodies.

These play a very prominent part in both protection against infection and in recovery once it has become active in the body. They are found in the fluid portion of the circulating blood and consist of a highly specialized form of protein known as immune globulin. They possess two important properties. They can bring about the destruction of microbes by various methods that do not need description or they can neutralize the toxins or poisons they produce.

Because of these activities, it was postulated soon after the discovery of the part played by microbes in the production of disease, that during most of our lives we succeed in remaining free of infection because we possess what are called natural antibodies that enable us to combat all the many microbes we encounter. But if for some reason these antibodies are deficient in quantity or quality, we then become infected.

Once infection has started, a second mechanism then comes into operation. Chemical substances, commonly called antigens, are released by the infecting microbes and are carried in the blood stream to the antibody-forming cells. The latter are thereby stimulated to produce more antibodies to make up the deficiency in natural antibodies. But in bringing this about the microbes encompass their own destruction because the new antibodies are carried to the infected area by the blood where they act in such a manner that the microbes are killed and their toxins neutralized. Theoretically, therefore, the patient should immediately start to recover. But if the antibodies are not produced, or only in an insufficient amount, the microbes get the upper hand and the patient dies. All this is of course an over-simplification, but for many years it was the standard doctrine of immunity.

If, then, recovery depends on the presence of antibodies in the blood stream, one form of treatment would obviously be to give them to the patient. It is possible to do this because they can be produced by giving animals a number of injections of killed microbes or the toxins they produce when growing in liquid medium. Although it ought, theoretically, to be possible to cure any infection by such antibodies, the facts, like so much that concerns immunity, do not always fit the theory. In one particular instance they do: this is diphtheria. Administration of the antitoxin can undoubtedly cure the disease. But although there may have been a few recoveries when antibodies have been used for the treatment of other diseases such as pneumonia, they have, on the whole, proved to be virtually useless.

Other methods of treatment by immunological methods were accordingly devised. They all rested on the assumption that when infection occurs, and so long as it continues to be active, it is primarily due to the fact that the patient cannot produce the antibodies required to cure himself. One of the most persistent advocates of this doctrine was Wright himself. His whole reasoning was based on a test known as the opsonic index, to which I will refer in more detail later, but which seemed to confirm his belief in this doctrine. He therefore advocated, and Wright could be a powerful advocate, the injection of small quantities of killed microbes or vaccines to stimulate further the antibody-forming cells. This method of treatment became known as vaccine therapy and was used a great deal before the First World War. But although the reasoning behind it seemed valid at the time, the method was, for all practical prurpose, useless.

Wright put forward another method of treatment after the war. It was founded on the assumption that the white cells in the circulating blood would, when stimulated by a vaccine, produce hitherto undetected antibodies which they released into the blood. This was based on experiments with a piece of apparatus known as a slide cell. The phenomenon detected in this way was known round the laboratory as 'immunity in vitro' and it led to the use of blood obtained from a suitable donor, adding the vaccine to it, and then administering it to the patient. Immuno-transfusion, as this method was called, was also found to be useless.

I had heard a great deal about these theories and the treatment that resulted from them when Wright lectured on immunity to the medical students. Being one of the best and most convincing lecturers I have ever heard, he had succeeded in conveying the impression that the theories were no longer theories, they were facts, and that any failures in treatment were due to something else, possibly lack of skill on the part of the doctor or even lack of co-operation on the part of the patient's immunity apparatus. Following advocacy of this type, it is perhaps not surprising that I had determined to serve under his banner. And when Colebrook found, soon after I started to work with him, that I could be trusted to handle dangerous microbes, he suggested that I investigate the immunity of patients with puerperal fever caused by highly virulent haemolytic streptococci, I naturally grasped the opportunity to confirm the theories of my hero.

Within a year I had made what were to me two shattering discoveries. The first was that none of the patients, no matter how severe their infection, was lacking in antibodies capable of dealing with these microbes. Whatever Wright had postulated, they had more than I myself or any other normal person possessed. In consequence, even when they were dying with enormous numbers of streptococci in the circulating blood, it could kill many more of these organisms than could mine. Something was obviously very wrong with the theory.

The second and in the circumstances much more dangerous discovery was that neither the opsonic index nor the slide cell methods Wright had used to prove his theories had been in any way adequate for the purpose. Since this is all past history it is unnecessary to go into details, but whatever the opsonic index measured it was certainly not the antibody level of the blood. It was more probably the erythrocyte sedimentation rate which has nothing to do with the killing of microbes. As for the slide cell, it was so inaccurate that the minute differences on which the theory of immunity in vitro depended were no more than the inherent experimental errors of the method.

What made this discovery so dangerous was that Wright considered himself to be a master of technique; so much so that he had published a book on the subject as long before as 1912 in which the method for determining the opsonic index had been described in minute detail.[76] The slide cell, too, had been described in a paper of such inordinate length that it had required no less than three instalments in the *Lancet* when it appeared in 1923.[78] Had I thrown such doubts on these techniques before the war I have no doubt that I would have been summarily dismissed, for he never allowed opposition within the camp at that time. I was, therefore, extremely nervous when I had to submit my work before publication. But I need not have worried. By this time Wright was no more than a shadow of his former self. He even congratulated me on it.

Thus, within a year of my starting to work with Colebrook it had become obvious that whatever was responsible for the patient becoming infected in the first place and for her death if the infection was severe, it was certainly not because of her inability to produce what apeared to be the most important antibodies. The vast edifice of theory erected by Wright which had led him to advocate treatment by vaccine therapy and immuno-transfusion had evidently rested on the most unstable of foundations.

Nevertheless, antibodies are not the only factors involved in immunity. Shortly before my arrival on the scene, it had been found that if the fat-soluble vitamin A was deficient in the diet, exposed tissues such as the eye or throat might become infected. There was also a notion, one could not call it evidence, that if the diet of a pregnant woman had been deficient, she was more likely to become infected after delivery of the baby. Prof. E. J. Mellanby and Dr C. N. Green of Sheffield accordingly assumed that puerperal fever might be due to a deficiency of vitamin A and used it to obtain a much higher proportion of recoveries than had anyone else.

The Department could not ignore this intrusion into its territory and a supply of the vitamin was obtained in a great hurry. The Sister in charge of the ward was told to administer it to a patient who had just been admitted with puerperal fever. It was not very long before she appeared in the laboratory with the information that the patient could not continue with the treatment. The taste was too horrible. This seemed to augur well for the future because it was still thought at that time that the worse the flavour the better the medicine. But to reassure her, I put a drop of the repulsive black oil on my tongue. Within seconds, my whole system seemed to be permeated with all the bad fish ever thrown overboard from a Grimsby trawler during a heat-wave. No matter what I did I could not get rid of it. Gargling, hot and cold drinks, not to mention spitting, all failed to dislodge it. In the end I had recourse to chewing gum, but even so it was a long time before the bad fish finally left me.

It would obviously have to be given in gelatin capsules, but the manufacturers could not supply them. The machine was too big to handle the small quantities we required. We accordingly obtained empty capsules from the dispensary and I proceeded to fill them. Although priding myself on my manual dexterity it was almost impossible to avoid some of the foul substance contaminating the outside in the process. And even if I got it inside safely, it showed a lamentable tendency to leak out before the capsule was finally swallowed. As the unfortunate patient had to have one every hour, I spent most of the next few days keeping ahead of her requirements.

All this might have been worth the trouble had she benefited. She did not. Nor did subsequent patients treated by this method. Whatever had cured the patients in Sheffield, it cannot have been vitamin A. Perhaps the clinicians in Sheffield had been too pessimistic about the chances of their patients and they would have recovered in any case.

No other immunological methods being forthcoming, even the collective wisdom of the Inoculation Department had to admit defeat.

A second and much older method of treatment was the administration of chemical compounds generally known as antiseptics such as carbolic acid, mercury perchloride and hypochlorous acid. This had been seriously considered as soon as the connection between microbes and disease had been established. It was no more than the logical outcome of the observation that compounds of this nature could kill microbes and sometimes in high dilution. Why not use them for the treatment of infections caused by them?

This, too, had not escaped the attention of the Inoculation Department largely because compounds of this nature had been employed a great deal for the treatment of infected wounds. It had come to a head during the early months of the First World War when the surgeons were faced with larger and more severely infected wounds than they had ever seen before. And it was largely because they had found that the antiseptics they used so lavishly were doing very little good that Wright and his men had been sent to Boulogne to investigate the matter.

In a series of extremely elegant experiments, they soon showed that the application of antiseptics to infected wounds was almost bound to fail for three reasons. Firstly, because antiseptics are quickly quenched by the body fluids and soon become useless. Secondly, they not only injure the body cells in the neighbourhood of the wound but, of more importance, the cells known as phagocytes that are responsible for repelling the invaders; and thirdly, because they probably fail to penetrate deep enough into the tissues to reach the microbes.[77]

If there was little justification for the treatment of open and accessible infections by antiseptics, there was even less for their use when the microbes were deep in the tissues causing infections such as septicaemia, pneumonia, meningitis and peritonitis. Not only would the same objections apply but there was also serious risk that any antiseptic injected into the blood stream, the only satisfactory method of ensuring that it reached the microbes, would poison the patient without necessarily harming the microbes. But despite all this, they were still being used in this way; so much so that Fleming once burst out with 'There are at least seven hospitals in London and Mary's is one of 'em, where they are regularly injecting this or that antiseptic into the blood stream in cases of septicaemia.'

Even when they were administered by less drastic methods than intravenous injection, there was no reason to suppose that would have much value. But in spite of this most medical wards smelled strongly of creosote, inhaled from a mask over their nose and mouth by patients with tuberculosis. The cresols in the inspired air were supposed to kill the tubercle bacilli in their lungs. I often wondered how many poor devils were hastened to their end by the combined effects of partial asphyxia and strong-smelling vapours.

Efforts were also being made to find antiseptics that would be poisonous for microbes but less poisonous for human beings than those usually employed. One of them was Mercurochrome, a mercury compound which was being used extensively in America. Although its sponsors were distinguished clinicians, they must have been advised by bacteriologists of singular incompetence. For, soon after my entry into chemotherapeutic research, Lord Balfour went to America and contracted a sore throat. He was given Mercurochrome to gargle and the sore throat disappeared. As he was, at that time, Lord President of the Council in which capacity he had to answer in Parliament for the deeds and misdeeds of the Medical Research Council, he summoned Sir Walter Fletcher, its secretary, and suggested that it should pay more attention to this new wonder drug that had so miraculously relieved him of his affliction. Fletcher naturally referred the problem to his chemotherapeutic expert, Colebrook. The latter then handed it to me. As there was no one lower in the scale to hand it to, I had to do the work.

It did not take very long to show that whatever had cured the eminent statesman's throat, it could not have been the Mercurochrome for it seemed singularly ineffective even in the test tube and still more so in the tissues. This is but one example of compounds of this nature that are, even now, used for the treatment of sore throats and colds. It is very doubtful whether they do any good. But one thing is quite certain, they cannot be classed as chemotherapeutic agents.

The third method of treatment was by what we know as chemotherapeutic substances such as the sulphonamides and antibiotics. Many years were to elapse before these compounds appeared but their precursors were already in existence. The first step in their evolution had been the discovery that atoxyl, an arsenical compound, could be used for the treatment of a disease of mice caused by spirochaetes. Ehrlich, the father of chemotherapy, hoped to use it for the treatment of syphilis which is also caused by spirochaetes but could not do so because it causes blindness when given to human beings. He then assumed that if the molecule of atoxyl was altered it might become less harmful for the patient and even more powerful in its effect on the microbe. Then began one of the most remarkable pieces of research in all bacteriology: the synthesis of compound after compound in the hope of producing one with the required properties. In the process there were no less than 605 failures, but the 606th was a success. For this reason, it was frequently known as '606' although its official name was Salvarsan or Arsphenamine.

It was far from ideal as a chemotherapeutic agent for it was so dangerous that only one dose could be administered every 7 days. To make matters worse, the drug itself in the form of a dry powder had to be dissolved, literally at the bedside, in no less than 600 c.c. of water. It was then given intravenously and if much escaped into the tissues round the vein, necrosis occurred that might lead to loss of the arm. Rashes might also develop and the liver be so damaged that the patient went yellow with jaundice. Treatment of this degree of ferocity generally went on for a year and sometimes more before the patient could be regarded as cured. Some of the dangers were eliminated when a second compound, Neosalvarsan – the 914th in the series – was synthesized, but prolonged treatment was still necessary.[22]

Introduced into medicine in 1910, these were the first synthetically produced compounds to have any real value for the treatment of a bacterial infection. The Inoculation Department had not been slow to appreciate their value, if only because Ehrlich, who was a great friend of Wright's, had sent him samples soon after their production. The latter had handed them to Fleming who became, in this way, one of the leading veneriologists in London before the war.

Except for two other spirochaetal infections, yaws and relapsing fever, it had not been suspected that such compounds would have much value for other forms of infection, but in 1911 it was observed that when they were used for the treatment of patients with syphilitic ulcers and skin eruptions which had become secondarily infected by staphylococci or streptococci, they healed as rapidly as those that had not been infected in this way. This suggested that the arsenicals might have chemotherapeutic activity on these organisms as well as on the spirochaetes. Having found that they could kill these organisms in the test tube, Colebrook, and Douglas, who was also a member of Wright's staff at that time, hoped to use them for the treatment of the severe infections of gunshot wounds that were so common in the base hospitals of France during the war. They were unable to do so because the war ended about this time.

When Colebrook returned to St Mary's after the war and became not only a member of the staff of the Medical Research Council but its – and in fact the country's – only expert on bacterial chemotherapy, he started to study these compounds in more detail. In order to assess their clinical value for streptococcal infections, he needed patients. Those with wounds infected to the same extent as those he had seen in France were too few in the hospitals of London. A suitable alternative was forthcoming in the form of puerperal fever. This is a severe infection following childbirth that is almost never seen nowadays but which, at that time, caused the death of two or even more women out of every thousand who had had a baby. Most of these infections were caused by exactly the same streptococci that had infected the wounds in France.

Colebrook accordingly began to study this disease and the possible use of the arsenicals for its treatment. He therefore spent much of his time, muffled up in a large raincoat, driving an open Morris Oxford car to the fever hospitals in Clapham and Hampstead to which many of the patients had been sent.

It was at this stage that I started to work with him. The arsenical compound he was using seemed to possess all the qualities required of a chemotherapeutic agent. When given by injection, sufficient quantities reached the circulating blood to render it capable of killing large numbers of haemolytic streptococci similar to those causing the infection. Nor did it injure the leucocytes, the main defensive mechanism of the body for dealing with microbes. Unfortunately, it was so poisonous that it was necessary to wait several days before another dose could be given. This was a serious hindrance but before very long Dr Ewins, a mild and gentle chemist from May and Baker, the pharmaceutical chemists, appeared in the laboratory with a sample of another compound called Metarsenobillon which was so much less poisonous that daily doses could be given. It was, moreover, equally efficient as that we had been using when tested *in vitro*.[9]

Colebrook did a great deal of work with this compound. I never counted the number of patients who received it but it must have been at least a hundred. Moreover, every case was studied with great care and a post-mortem was done if the patient died. Variations were made in the dosage and every trick that might have given it a better chance was tried. But I am quite certain that we never cured a patient by giving it. So far as I could see it was a total failure.

I realized this quite early in the proceedings. Colebrook did not and went on using it. But it meant that I had to lie like a trooper when asked by puzzled clinicians why we persisted in using a drug that was obviously doing no good.

Such then was the position in the year or two following my starting to work with Colebrook. No immunological method of treatment, no matter how brilliantly argued, evidently had a chance against severe streptococcal or similar infections; antiseptics were more likely to do harm than good; the only chemotherapeutic compounds of any value were the arsenicals and although they could cure syphilis, they obviously could not cure streptococcal infections. Perhaps this may explain why half the Medical Research Council's only unit for the study of streptococcal infection in general, and its chemotherapy in particular, consisted of one recently qualified and almost untrained Licentiate of the Society of Apothecaries.

Although none of us knew it, this was but the deeper darkness that precedes the dawn. Before 1928 was out, the most important of the substances that eventually solved the problem had been found. This was penicillin, discovered by Alexander Fleming working only a few feet away on the floor below.

Chapter 3

The Discovery of Penicillin

Towards the end of August 1928, I came back from a holiday with Dr D. M. Pryce and resumed the task of demolishing the *bona fides* of the opsonic index, a matter which still seemed to be of paramount medical importance. In those days the time-wasting custom of morning coffee and gossip had not been invented; at least, it was not the custom in the Inoculation Department. But we still wasted our time by gossiping. Fleming was no exception and in order to do so had to leave his little room down the staircase to find someone with whom to gossip. He had, therefore, evolved the custom of indulging in a morning potter which included a visit to the big laboratory in which I was working.

Fleming's idea of gossip was different from that of most other people. It usually involved his planting himself in front of the fireplace with his hands in his pockets, a cigarette dangling from his lips and looking more or less into space. On rare occasions he would give utterance, usually in the fewest possible words. The information doled out so meagrely might concern anything; that so-and-so had died; that what's-his-name had made a fool of himself again; or how are your Snia Viscosa's doing? This would be addressed to Hayden who, with Fleming, steadily lost money – or so it seemed to the rest of us – on shares whose purchase had been strongly recommended by the third financial wizard in the Department, Matthews. He, it appeared, was frequently given inside information by the peers and big business men who formed the bulk of his practice.

On this occasion it was neither Fleming's notion of gossip nor high finance that emerged. It was the now famous culture plate that led to the discovery of penicillin. The rest of us, being engaged in researches that seemed far more important than a contaminated culture plate, merely glanced at it, thought that it was no more than another wonder of nature that Fleming seemed to be forever unearthing, and promptly forgot all about it.

The plate was also shown to Wright when he arrived in the afternoon. What he said, I do not recollect, but since Wright was seldom enthusiastic about anything that did not concern logic or immunity in vitro, one can assume that he was no more enthusiastic – he could not have been less – than the rest of us had been that morning.

Unfortunately we were not allowed to forget the plate altogether. It began to make its presence felt in the laboratory. Dr S. R. Craddock, who had become a Research Scholar and was working with Fleming, seemed to spend a great deal of his time cherishing bottles or flasks containing a bright yellow fluid which he told us was mould juice. This did not matter very much; in fact it imparted a little colour into our drab lives. He and Mr F. Ridley, a young ophthalmologist who was also working with Fleming, then started to do what seemed to the rest of us somewhat amateurish experiments of a chemical nature in the narrow passage outside our laboratory. This did not matter either. If they wanted to get pneumonia by standing about in the draught it was their business. But what did upset all of us was that they seriously impeded our excursions to the only lavatory on the floor, which happened to be on the further side of their chemical activities, and to get there usually meant asking them to get out of the way. For they were both big men.

When the warmer weather came in the spring, and with it less risk of their catching colds, their activities in the passage ceased. Nor were we reminded of them on the rare occasions when Fleming gave utterance at the tea-table. And by the time I went on holiday again, I had forgotten all about Fleming's contaminated culture plate.

Such then was what I saw of the discovery of penicillin and its aftermath. The events that led up to it, the manner in which the discovery was made, the properties of the substance, all were described in what is now a classical paper which was published in June 1929.[24] After Fleming's death, accounts also appeared in the many obituary notices that were written by his friends and colleagues.[2, 11, 17] And finally, in 1959, there appeared the English translation by Gerard Hopkins of his biography, written by André Maurois, the distinguished French novelist and biographer.[63]

Evidently basing their accounts on what Fleming wrote or said on many occasions, all these authors describe the discovery of penicillin as the result of a chance observation of a comparatively common event in bacteriological laboratories: contamination of a culture plate by air-borne moulds and microbes while it is opened for inspection. They must have also assumed, if only because they say virtually nothing about it, that as the particular variety of mould is a common species, its source and the processes by which it reached the plate can have been of no particular importance.

If these assumptions had been justified, nothing further need be said; but when, in 1964, sufficient leisure became available to enable me to make the necessary enquiries and carry out essential laboratory investigations, it became only too obvious that the history of both the culture plate and the mould itself must have been very different from what had previously been thought to be the case. In fact, so much so, that far from the phenomenon that led to the discovery being a comparatively common event that had previously escaped detection, it must be so unusual an occurrence that it is doubtful whether it can have happened very often since bacteria were first cultivated in the laboratory.

The events that followed the discovery were also described by the authors referred to above but, for no very obvious reason, a great deal of important work carried out by Fleming and his assistants was either omitted or inadequately described. An attempt was also made to explain the inescapable fact that Fleming never demonstrated the value of penicillin as a chemotherapeutic agent. In doing so, excuses were put forward whose validity is doubtful, and his biographer even goes so far as to make accusations of deliberate obstruction.

Thus the existing accounts of both the discovery of penicillin and its aftermath cannot be described as satisfactory. But largely because the discovery was probably one of the most important scientific events of this century, I propose to describe what I know of it in considerable detail in this and the following three chapters.

Before embarking on this I must say something about the personality of the chief actor, if only because personality plays a much more important part in research than is usually realized. At the time he discovered penicillin Fleming was only 47 years old. Invariably referred to as Flem., he was small, with blue eyes, a large head, a bent nose and a broad Ayrshire accent. Unlike his colleagues he had come from a poor home. The son of a farmer in the Scottish lowlands, he had worked for a time as a clerk in a city office. He only succeeded in taking up medicine because someone left him some money. Although he took the Fellowship of the Royal College of Surgeons soon after obtaining his London degree, he never practised as a surgeon. Instead, he became a member of Wright's team almost at once, went to France with him during the First World War, and remained with him until he died. So far as I know, he never made any attempt to find another job. He was appointed Professor of Bacteriology in the University of London in 1928, and was assistant director of the Inoculation Department from the end of the First World War until Wright retired in 1945, when he succeeded him as Director of the Wright–Fleming Institute.

As a young man he had taken part in all the nocturnal activities of the department and worked as hard as any of them. But by the time I got to known him he had settled down to a comparatively blameless and contented existence which involved nothing more exciting than life in a Chelsea flat in the ground floor and basement of a Victorian villa in Danvers Street, between the art shops of the King's Road and the half lights of Whistler's Thames at Battersea Bridge. But practically every week-end and all his holidays were spent at a country house near Newmarket where he cultivated a garden and fished in the river at the bottom of it. The nearest he got to excitement was a visit to the Chelsea Arts Club on the way from the laboratory, before going home to dinner. Here he met most of the well-known artists to whom he seemed to act as a sort of honorary medical adviser; not, perhaps, completely honorary, because they gave him pictures in return and his flat became a miniature picture gallery with representative works by Philip Connard, Wilson Steer and Ronald Grey in particular.

He seemed to be reasonably well off. Except for the legacy that put him through medicine, I doubt whether he inherited money from his family. But I think he made a lot of money before the First World War by treating patients with syphilis. Not only was he one of the first to use the new drug '606' (Salvarsan), but he was one of the few who could be trusted to give it safely. After the war, he no longer did this but made vaccines for some of the physicians. Little was said about this activity but I think it brought him quite a large income. And although he received a salary from the Department, his manner of life was far beyond what this can have brought him.

It was possibly because of this security, following his impecunious beginnings, that he had become so settled in his habits. He was not lazy, but he was never in a hurry. He arrived every morning on the stroke of nine and departed punctually at five. Although taciturn, he liked company. If there was a party to go to, he went and enjoyed himself. He attended all the scientific meetings, mostly to meet other people. He and his wife also entertained a great deal. They held a large party during the Second International Congress of Microbiology in London and, quite spontaneously, he took about six of us to dinner at the Arts Club for no other reason than that we were all going to a lecture by Wright at the Pharmaceutical Society.

He was also a regular attendant at football matches and boxing and shooting competitions. He could, quite happily, spend hours at auction sales acquiring lots of very doubtful value. Whole days might be spent with such trophies. Once it was a telescope he set up on the roof of the laboratory to look at the London skyline. I myself profited by these excursions, for he gave me quite a respectable set of golf clubs picked up at auctions.

Although apparently so casual and, to some, even lazy, he

was in actual fact the catalyst who made the Department function. Wright was quite incapable of dealing with the petty details of administration and left almost everything to Fleming. But he had plenty of time to do research.

Nor did he lack assistance. It is true that he did not have the services of a trained technician – none of us did, it was contrary to the traditions of the laboratory – but he had what was much better, at least one and sometimes two young doctors who were prepared to work much harder. Following the First World War, Dr V. D. Allison worked for three years with him while holding a Beit Memorial Fellowship and played an important part in the study of lysozyme. Then came D. M. Pryce, and at the time of the discovery of penicillin he had two assistants, Frederick Ridley and Stuart Craddock. C. E. Dolman followed until he left for Canada in 1931. The next, K. B. Rogers, stayed until the war broke out. Mention must also be made of I. H. Maclean who shared his laboratory for several years and L. B. Holt who came in 1934 and remained on the staff until quite recently. These are only a few of the young men who worked with him during what might be called the penicillin period.

Even without his discovery of penicillin, Fleming would have left his mark on bacteriology. His methods for the staining of spores and flagella are still used. He was one of the first to identify the organisms that cause infection of wounds and must have been the very first to show that cross-infection by streptococci can occur in hospital wards. He also studied in very considerable detail the effect of antiseptics on microbes and living tissues. But I have no doubt that he himself thought that his most solid contribution was the discovery of lysozyme.[28] This is a ferment present in tears, nasal mucus and saliva, that kills and dissolves almost at once most of the microbes that reach these surfaces from the atmosphere. It is a very striking experiment to put a drop of tears on to a colony of one of these organisms and watch it disappear under one's eyes. Of equal, if not greater importance, is the fact that lysozyme does not confine its activities to human beings or even animals; it is present in the eggs of birds and fishes and can also be found in seeds of all kinds. It is, therefore, what one might call a universal biological protective mechanism for preventing microbes from destroying the means of reproduction and the areas of the body that are most exposed to microbes in the environment.

If such a substance is not physiologically and bacteriologically of great importance, I do not know what is. But, unfortunately for Fleming, its action on organisms that cause disease is less obvious. I say 'unfortunately' because at that time, and even now, all that most medical bacteriologists care about are microbes that cause disease. Few think beyond disease and realize that there are other microbes that are of equal if not greater importance. And so Fleming's fundamental discovery, for it was all of that, lay completely neglected until someone found that lysozyme was present in leucocytes, that is to say, the white cells of the blood. It then became respectable and worthy of study. But even now it merits only a small paragraph in the larger textbooks.

Much of the neglect by others of lysozyme and to an even greater extent of penicillin was due, I think, to Fleming's inability to express himself clearly and lucidly in either words or print. He was certainly one of the worst lecturers I have ever heard. It cannot have been due to shyness because, so far as I know, he never refused an invitation to speak in public and he must have given hundreds of lectures and speeches after he became famous. In a dull monotone, without humour or emphasis, they may have given the audience the facts but that is about the best that can be said for them. His papers, too, gave the facts but little more. Prolixity, at which Wright was an adept, should it is true be avoided, but Fleming went to the other extreme and was much too economical with words.

I strongly suspect that the underlying cause of this was that he had such bacteriological green fingers that his experiments were planned and carried out more by instinct than thought. It probably never occurred to him that others would be unable to divine how he did them and how he reached his conclusions. The paper that describes the discovery of penicillin, for example, omits so much that it is quite impossible to repeat many of his experiments in the way he did them. Knowing him and his methods, one can guess what he had done, but no one else could.

He was equally uninformative in his speeches. I well remember an occasion when he spoke on lysozyme to an audience of medical men who knew very little bacteriology. He not only failed to tell them what the substance is, but where it comes from and its importance. About the only thing they gathered after half an hour was that lysozyme could evidently kill an organism of which they had never heard.

Much of this was, I am certain, due to the fact that what mattered most to Fleming was not the recording of his experiments but their performance. It may seem strange that I should have said this because most scientists do experiments. It is an important part of their daily lives. But it is the result of the experiment that matters to them. So it did to Fleming, but this was a secondary consideration. It was the actual performance of the experiment that he loved.

All his techniques were micro-methods stemming from those Wright had invented for his own work on the immunity mechanisms. Since the tests were carried out with human blood which had to be taken at frequent intervals, they had to be adapted for the use of very small quantities of reagents. Nor were they elaborate, requiring little more than glass tubing, teats, microscope slides, paraffin wax, Vaseline and plasticine. Although all of us used these methods and generally invented the actual techniques we used, none of us got the pleasure from this that Fleming did. He quite literally delighted in the invention of techniques and in the performance of the experiments he did with them.

In this respect he was poles apart from Florey, who worked in what was fundamentally the same type of laboratory but employed very different methods, in the experiments that finally proved the value of penicillin as a chemotherapeutic agent. Merely to produce sufficient penicillin for the treatment of small animals such as mice, he had to invoke the assistance of no less than six colleagues and many technicians who produced mould juice by the gallon in containers originally intended for use as bedpans. It was then purified by Chain in an apparatus as far removed in size from the pipettes and test tubes that sufficed for Fleming as the Empire State Building is from a lakeside cottage in Vermont. Small wonder that Fleming never got very far in his attempts to purify penicillin.

He was also very different from everyone else in his own laboratory. Wright looked on research as an intellectual exercise and used experiments to prove to lesser men, conclusions he had reached as a result of sheer cerebration. The experiment itself was a nuisance that had, unfortunately, to be performed for the sake of scientific convention. Colebrook did experiments because he was, fundamentally, a reformer who wanted to save humanity from its ills. For this reason, he was the one really dedicated scientist in the place. But all his experiments were strictly utilitarian, no more than a means to an end, the eradication of the particular disease he was interested in at the moment.

Such then, is something about the man who discovered penicillin. The process that led to it started soon after the First World War when Fleming began to hold a clinic for the treatment of patients with boils. Although it is doubtful whether the administration of vaccines, which was all he could do, can have been of much value, he became one of the few bacteriologists to take much interest in the staphylococci responsible for them. Strange as it may seem, in view of the importance with which it is nowadays regarded, this microbe was almost completely ignored in 1928. Any bacteriologist who wanted to get on in the world confined his attentions to more lethal microbes such as streptococci and pneumococci.

In view of the fact that staphylococci played an important part in the discovery of penicillin, it may be as well if I describe them in a little more detail. They are spherical particles about 1/1,000 mm. in diameter, and when seen down the microscope do not assume any particular pattern. There are two varieties: one, known as *Staphylococcus albus*, produces pure white colonies when growing on agar. Although present on all our skins, it seldom causes infection. The other, *Staphylococcus aureus* produces buff-yellow colonies and is much more important. Besides boils it causes carbuncles and a severe infection of the bones, now rare, called osteomyelitis. It may also infect wounds and produce infections of the fingers and hand called whitlows. Although painful and sometimes mutilating, such infections seldom cause death.

Because of his knowledge of this organism, Fleming was the obvious choice for the authorship of the chapter describing it in the large nine-volume *System of Bacteriology* which was being published about that time by the Medical Research Council. A composite work, each section being written by an expert, it was generally referred to in the laboratory as 'the Bible' because it was supposed to embody the whole of existing knowledge. Perhaps its most useful function, even if not anticipated by its editors, was that late in 1927 while writing his chapter, Fleming read a paper by Bigger, Boland and O'Meara of Trinity College, Dublin, in which it was stated that under certain circumstances, colonies of staphylococci on solid media may be different in a number of respects, chiefly their colour, from those usually produced.[4] Fleming considered it necessary to study these variants. In this, he had been helped by D. M. Pryce, a Research Scholar, but in February, 1928, the latter accepted a post under Prof. Newcomb in the Department of Pathology.

Fleming carried on with the work himself. It involved growing the microbes on culture plates. These are shallow glass dishes known as petri dishes in the bottom of which is a thin layer of a gelatinous substance called agar containing enough nutrients to enable the microbes to multiply when placed on the surface. The process of cultivation is extremely simple because all that it involves is spreading a small number of the microbes over the surface of the agar with a platinum wire and then incubating the plate at a suitable temperature which is generally 98·6°F (37°C) for 16–24 hours. The microbes multiply so rapidly that they form masses or colonies that are easily visible at the end of that time.

A great deal of useful information can be obtained merely by examining the colour, size and general appearance of the colonies. And it was for this particular purpose that Fleming was using these plates. When it is necessary to study the organisms further, some are taken from one of the colonies on a platinum wire, spread over the surface of a fresh plate, and incubated in turn. As a result of this, quite large numbers of such plates may be used. Most workers discard them as soon as possible but Fleming tended to hoard his on his bench until he was quite certain that he no longer required them.

In the midst of this, towards the end of July or the beginning of August, Fleming took his family away for the summer holiday to his country house near Newmarket. Before doing so, he piled the plates that were by this time taking up much too much room on his bench, out of the way in the far, right-hand corner of the laboratory where the sun could not reach them.[16] This provided space for S. R. Craddock, who had been recently recruited as a Research Scholar to replace Pryce and was to work in Fleming's laboratory during his absence, so that I. H. Maclean, another temporary occupant, could keep an eye on him.

When therefore, Fleming returned in September from his holiday, he was faced with these piles of plates. He began to go over them, making subcultures of the strains he wished to preserve. The old plates were then discarded. In a properly organized laboratory, this would have involved their being plunged into buckets of antiseptic such as lysol in which they would have been totally submerged. The organisms would have been killed at once and so made the glassware safe enough for the technicians to wash and prepare for use again. But at that time the Inoculation Department, probably because of its love for micro-methods, did not employ anything so big or so efficient as buckets. It made use of shallow enamel trays containing so little antiseptic that it was only possible to submerge about half a dozen petri dishes at a time. Any more to be discarded had to be piled up on top.

Fleming's lysol tray seems to have reached this stage when Pryce, following his holiday with me, came to see him early in September. Fleming looked up from his work and, pointing to the piles of discarded plates, remarked that they were the result of Pryce's desire to become a morbid anatomist. He, Fleming, was now having to do all the work himself, and look how his bench had become cluttered. Nevertheless, Pryce was sufficiently interested in the work to ask for details. To demonstrate a point, Fleming took the plates standing high and dry on top of the pile in the lysol tray, which he had evidently inspected already and then discarded, to show him the colonies.[67] There were moulds and yeasts on them as well as the colonies of staphylococci, but nothing that was unusual. Except that one of these plates was unusual. Pryce told me long afterwards what happened. 'He took the plate up, looked at it, and after a while said, "That's funny".' This was the now famous plate that demonstrated the ability of penicillin coming from a colony of a mould to act on staphylococci in its vicinity. They discussed the probable reasons for what they had seen, agreed that it was extremely abnormal, and the discussion ended with Fleming making a subculture of the mould into a tube of broth.

The plate was then shown to anyone handy. One of the first must have been E. W. Todd, just back from a year at the Rockefeller Institute in New York, who was the other occupant of Fleming's laboratory for several more years. All he could say was that it was very interesting; but in spite of this lack of enthusiasm at the time, claimed in after years that if Fleming went to the House of Lords he, Todd, ought to have a knighthood.

Shortly after this Dr Hurst Brown, a Canadian Rhodes Scholar, visited Fleming and was duly shown the plate with the remark, 'You think yourself a clever fellow, explain this one'. Another caller was Dr C. J. La Touche, the mycologist from the floor below. He too expressed interest in a mould that was doing something unusual but did not then realize, as I shall suggest in the next chapter, that he had a proprietary interest in the mould on the plate. The plate was then, as I have already related, shown to the unappreciative audience in the laboratory upstairs and to Wright when he arrived in the afternoon.

I think it would be true to say that everyone who has thought seriously about the discovery has assumed that what Fleming saw that September morning is a comparatively common event, but which had not been noticed before because bacteriologists had been too myopic to see it and, even if they had, had been too incurious to do anything about it. In actual fact the real story must be very different. The phenomenon that led to the discovery of penicillin can only be reproduced when certain special and somewhat unusual requirements are met. So much is this so that it is very doubtful whether it can have occurred more than a very few times since bacteriologists first started to cultivate microbes on culture plates.

Let us start by considering exactly what Fleming showed Pryce that morning. A photograph of the plate was evidently taken but prints are no longer available. The best that can be done is to reproduce the half-tone plate in the original paper. It suffices to illustrate the principal features, and if it is assumed that its diameter was the usual 85 mm., some idea of the measurements can also be obtained from an enlargement I had made. It shows what are evidently separate, well-grown colonies of staphylococci 2–4 mm. in diameter over most of the surface of the medium. But towards one edge of the plate there is a colony of the mould about 20 mm. in diameter, to which is attached a smaller satellite. Round it, in a zone about 20 mm. in width, there are either no visible colonies of the staphylococci or only tiny semi-transparent masses that can best be described as ghosts. There are about sixteen of them, those nearest to the mould being only 0·4–0·8 mm. in diameter while those towards the periphery are 0·8–1·7 mm.

All that is known about the history of the plate is what Fleming said in the original paper. It constitutes the opening paragraph and is as follows: 'While working with staphylococcal variants, a number of culture plates were set aside on the laboratory bench and examined from time to time. In the examinations, these plates were necessarily exposed to the air and they became contaminated with various micro-organisms. It was noticed that around a large colony of a contaminating mould, the staphylococcal colonies became transparent and were obviously undergoing lysis.'[24]

As a description of a scientific experiment or even an accidental observation, it leaves a great deal to be desired. He does not, for example, say what type of medium he was using; whether or not the plate had been incubated; how long it had been on the bench and perhaps the most remarkable omission of all, he does not even say what species of staphylococci he was studying. One must therefore resort to guess-work to describe the probable sequence of events that had led to the discovery. It was probably along the following lines.

Using a platinum wire, he had spread small numbers of staphylococci over the surface of an ordinary nutrient, agar culture plate and then incubated it at 98·6°F (37°C) for 16–24 hours, the usual time and temperature required for the production of colonies. The plate was then taken out of the incubator and left on the bench for some days or weeks. From time to time the colonies had been examined with a microscope to see whether they had undergone any change. While the plate was exposed in this way, airborne organisms and particularly the spores of moulds had reached the surface of the medium. Some of them had developed into colonies in the course of a few days. One of these colonies had produced penicillin which diffused through the agar round about; it attacked the normally opaque, yellowish colonies of staphylococci in the neighbourhood and, as a result, they underwent dissolution or lysis as it is usually called, into amorphous, transparent, watery masses. Colonies further removed remained unaltered.

Although he never actually said so, there seems little doubt that Fleming thought that this had been the sequence of events. He must therefore have assumed that before the spore reached the plate there had been fully developed colonies on the area round the mould colony that was subsequently found to be free of them. No other interpretation can be put on the statement in the original paper that 'the staphylococcal colonies became transparent and were obviously undergoing lysis',[24] and the use of the term 'degenerate colonies' to describe the ghosts, in a sketch reproduced in the biography.[63] Something in very similar vein was said on two subsequent occasions. Thus, in 1944 he went so far as to say, 'what had originally been a well-grown staphylococcal colony was now a faint shadow of its former self',[33] and in the Nobel Lecture of 1945, he said, 'the staphylococcal colonies had become translucent and evidently lysis was going on'.[36]

If this had been the sequence of events, penicillin would probably have been discovered while Fleming was still a child because contamination of culture plates by moulds is a comparatively common event in laboratories. But there are many reasons for supposing that the history of this culture plate was very different. The best way to demonstrate this is to attempt to 'discover' penicillin by this method. For this purpose I used Fleming's strain of the mould and the Oxford strain of staphylococci which is highly sensitive to the action of penicillin. I need not repeat exactly what I did because it was fundamentally as I have suggested above.

Taking an ordinary nutrient agar culture plate, I seeded it with staphylococci and incubated it at 98·6°F (37°C) for 24 hours. Fully developed, opaque, yellowish colonies had by that time been produced. Then, using a fine needle, a few spores of the mould were placed on the surface of the agar at a point where the colonies were well separated. The plate was then left on the bench and examined every day.

Much to my surprise, the mould which usually develops quite well at room temperature, its colonies reaching diameters of 8–10 mm. as early as the fourth day and 20 mm. after a fortnight, seemed very reluctant to grow. So unexpected was this that I investigated the matter in some detail. I soon found that whether or not the spores developed into a colony depended to a very large extent on the number and proximity of any staphylococcal colonies in the neighbourhood. If they were numerous and close to the spores, the latter generally failed to grow at all. Growth was more likely to occur if the colonies were fewer and some distance away; but, even when they did, the colony that was produced might reach a diameter of only 5–10 mm. before its further development was halted. No matter how long the plate was kept, it generally got no larger.

I then examined the photograph of Fleming's culture plate more closely and found that if the spores had reached the plate after the staphylococcal colonies had developed, there must have been about 200 such colonies on the plate, fairly evenly distributed over its surface. Furthermore, the spores must have reached its surface in close proximity to some of them if one assumes that the centre of the mould colony is the place where they had alighted. Under such conditions it is extremely improbable that the spores would have grown at all. And even if they had, it is also improbable that the colony produced would have become anything like the size of that on the plate which was not only 20 mm. in diameter but had even produced a small attached satellite as well.

In order to make certain of these conclusions, I carried out a great many experiments in which culture plates with approximately the same number of staphylococcal colonies as had been present on Fleming's plate were prepared and spores of the mould placed in much the same position as his mould colony. As I expected by now, they either failed to develop or the resulting colony was only about 10 mm. or even less in diameter.

I do not know why the proximity of fully developed colonies of staphylococci should prevent growth of the mould or bring it to a halt after it has started. One must presume that it is due to some soluble product coming from the organisms but it is improbable that it is acidity because the agar is alkaline when tested with litmus paper.

A mould colony will, however, develop if the spores reach the plate some distance from the staphylococcal colonies or there are only a few near the point of inoculation. In view of the number (200) and spacing of the colonies on Fleming's plate, it is just possible that the mould did reach the plate at a point where it could develop and produce penicillin. It was therefore necessary to ascertain whether it would have had any effect on the staphylococcal colonies in its vicinity. Experiments were accordingly carried out in which the mould was inoculated 10 mm. or more away from the nearest colonies and allowed to develop into a colony. But although its diameter might reach as much as 20 mm., the staphylococcal colonies remained completely unaffected no matter how long the plate was kept. No one looking at such a plate could possibly guess that a powerful antibacterial substance was emanating from the mould. I need hardly add that suitable control experiments, that need not be described, showed that penicillin was in fact being produced and was present in high concentration in the agar beneath the staphylococcal colonies.

In view of these experiments, it is extremely improbable that the mould spore can have reached the culture plate after the colonies of staphylococci had fully developed, partly because the mould would probably have failed to grow at all, and partly because if it did the penicillin produced would have had no visible effect on the staphylococcal colonies in its vicinity.

In regard to the second of these two conclusions, my friend Dr W. D. Foster has also found that penicillin from a developing mould colony has no action on fully developed colonies of staphylococci. But he went further and, to make quite certain that it was not due to lack of penicillin, dropped crystals of the drug on to the colonies so that its concentration in their vicinity must have been astronomical. But even treatment of this nature left them unaffected.

In 1944, long before either of us had thought of doing this, Dr Margaret Jennings (now Lady Florey) had similarly failed to show that penicillin from colonies of the mould had any effect on fully grown staphylococcal colonies.[54] Nor did a solution coming from cylinders (Heatley cups) on the surface of the medium. Thus one must conclude that penicillin, whether in the form of crystals, in solution, or coming from the mould itself, has no visible action on fully grown colonies of staphylococci.

Why this should be so was discovered as early as 1942 and has been confirmed on many occasions since that time. It is simply this: that penicillin can only act on microbes while they are young and actively multiplying. Synthesis of the mucopeptides that constitute the cell walls is brought to a halt, they become so weak that they give way and the organism bursts, releasing its contents into the surrounding medium in the form of an amorphous completely transparent watery mass. But penicillin has no such action on cells that are not multiplying or are incapable of multiplication because they have died of old age.[51]

A very high proportion of the staphylococci that make up a colony that has reached maturity are long past the stage in their life cycle at which penicillin can have any action on them. The very great majority are already dead, probably killed by the acids and other substances they produce in the course of growth. Only a very small minority will be multiplying or even capable of doing so. And even if penicillin in high concentration reaches such a colony, the dissolution of the few cells that are still capable of multiplication is unlikely to have any visible effect on the architecture of the colony. Because of this, it could have been predicted as long ago as 1942 that Lady Florey, Foster and myself would have obtained the results we did.

In view of this, it is extremely improbable that the history of Fleming's culture plate can have been what he or most commentators have assumed it to have been. The plate cannot have gone through what might be called the normal procedures involved in the cultivation of microbes or even the processes by which culture plates become contaminated. What then was its history?

Ignoring the assumptions Fleming seems to have made, all that is certain is that the plate had been on his bench for 4 or 5 weeks and that at the end of that time there were either no staphylococcal colonies or only ghosts in the vicinity of the mould. Is it not possible that the staphylococci had been attacked at a much earlier period in their life history when they were so young that a high proportion of the organisms in the developing colonies were still alive and multiplying? The effect of penicillin on such organisms can be devastating, for within a few hours practically all the organisms have undergone dissolution; the tiny but otherwise normal colony becomes transformed into a watery amorphous mass which is so completely transparent that it is only just visible on the surface of the medium when viewed by oblique illumination. Somewhat older colonies containing a higher proportion of organisms that have died undergo fundamentally the same alteration, but the dead organisms being unaffected by the penicillin become distributed throughout the mass to give it a whitish appearance, so that the colonies resemble drops of very dilute milk. Such is, undoubtedly, the causation of the ghosts in Fleming's photograph.

Innumerable experiments carried out since the discovery of penicillin have all shown that this is, undoubtedly, what had produced the phenomenon on the culture plate that led to its discovery. The staphylococci had, as Fleming said they had, undergone lysis, but it was not the lysis of those in relatively old fully mature colonies that had been the cause of the phenomenon.

It was the lysis of those in young colonies in an earlier stage of their development.

This provides a clue to the probable history of the culture plate for it shows that the mould must have developed into a colony which had begun to produce penicillin before any staphylococci on the plate had started to multiply. It is, therefore, very easy to 'discover' penicillin by putting spores of the mould on to a culture plate, allowing them to develop into a colony about 10 mm. in diameter, and then seeding the plate with staphylococci up to the margin of the mould. If the plate is then incubated or even left on the bench – it does not matter which – a picture almost indistinguishable from that of Fleming's original plate is produced. But penicillin cannot have been discovered in this way. No one uses a culture plate with a large colony of a mould already growing on it. Certainly not Fleming.

If, on the other hand, the mould spore reached the plate at the time, or within a few hours, of its being seeded with staphylococci, it might have been possible to discover penicillin if multiplication of the staphylococci could have been postponed until the mould had started to grow and produce penicillin. Although a whole series of factors would have played a part in bringing this about, the most important would have been the temperature because the speed of growth of the mould is not greatly affected over a wide range of temperatures, whereas that of the staphylococci certainly is; so much so that the lowest at which any growth occurs at all, and then only very slowly, is in the neighbourhood of 53°F (12°C) and the most rapid growth is at 98·6°F (37°C). It therefore seemed possible that the discovery might have been made if the plate had been kept at an intermediate level such as room temperature, so that growth of the staphylococci could have been delayed long enough to enable the mould to develop into a colony and produce penicillin, which would then act on the staphylococci in the vicinity before they became insusceptible.

On the offchance that something of this nature had been the underlying cause of the discovery, I set up an experiment on August 1, 1966 in which I inoculated an ordinary nutrient agar culture plate with the Oxford staphylococcus and planted a few spores of Fleming's strain of the mould on the plate at one spot. I then put the plate on the bench in the shade and inspected it every day thereafter. As I had expected, the staphylococci grew much more slowly than they would have done in an incubator. So much so that only tiny transparent colonies were visible on the third day. The mould, however, developed quite satisfactorily so that a tiny colony was already visible after 48 hours, reached 10 mm. in diameter on the fourth day, and 15 mm. on the sixth.

By the end of the fifth day it was obvious that I had rediscovered penicillin. The staphylococcal colonies in a zone about 10 mm. round the mould were still only pin-point in size and transparent, whereas those on more distant parts of the plate had become larger and more opaque. They were beginning to resemble those produced in only 24 hours in an incubator. As the days passed, the contrast between the two types of colony became even more marked. The general picture was indistinguishable from the photograph in Fleming's paper.

I was then foolish enough to repeat the experiment on August 15. I say foolish because it is generally inadvisable to repeat a successful experiment. This time I did not discover penicillin. Both the staphylococci and the mould grew quite satisfactorily but there was no sign whatever that anything coming from the mould was acting on the microbes. At first I was nonplussed by this failure, for so far as I knew I had followed exactly the same procedures. But close examination of the plates showed that the staphylococcal colonies had reached maturity much sooner than in the first experiment. This suggested that most of the organisms in them had become too old to be susceptible to penicillin before the mould had had time to grow and produce it.

Why this had occurred was soon determined because I had had the foresight to take the temperatures of the culture plates several times a day during both experiments. These records showed that during the first experiment, their temperature had been comparatively low, 61–65°F (16·1–18·3°C) the weather having been cold, wet and stormy. But during the second experiment the weather had become hot and sunny so that their temperature had been as high as 71–75°F (21·7–23·9°C).

It therefore seemed probable that my re-discovery of penicillin in early August had been due to the fortunate chance that the weather had been cold enough to retard growth of the staphylococci until the mould had grown enough to produce penicillin, and my failure in the middle of the month to the fact that the weather had become warmer and the staphylococci grew too quickly. Although it seemed odd that a difference of only about 6°C or 10°F could be so critical, I set up a more sophisticated experiment to find out whether such was really the case.

In this, I took three sets of culture plates and inoculated each of them with staphylococci in the usual way and then placed a few spores of the mould on each of them at one point. Then, by utilizing the central heating resources of a London flat (autumn had arrived by the time I started this experiment) I kept them at temperatures that ranged from the very hot to the coolest consistent with comfort. That is to say, one set at 98–99°F (36·6–36·2°C) by placing them over a radiator, another at 72–74°F (22·2–23·3°C) in the airing cupboard and a third in an unheated bedroom at 61–63°F (16–17·2°C). Despite this rather amateurish procedure there was very little fluctuation in the temperatures.

The plates were inspected every day and the results were exactly as I had expected. At 98–99°F the staphylococci on all the plates reached maturity and accordingly became insusceptible to penicillin long before the mould had even started to grow. Their rate of growth at 72–74°F was slower and although the the mould colonies had become 5, 4, 3, 2 and 1 mm. in diameter on the five plates after only three days, penicillin had evidently not been formed early enough to act on the staphylococci. Their colonies had become full-sized by this time. The mould colonies increased in diameter with the passage of time but nothing even remotely resembling Fleming's phenomenon could be seen on any of the plates.

On all the plates kept at 61–63°F, a very different picture was produced and almost indistinguishable from that on the plate I had set up on August 1 when the temperature had been much the same. The mould had evidently developed quickly enough and growth of the staphylococci had been retarded enough for the newly formed penicillin to prevent their further development.

In many subsequent experiments it was found that although it is nearly always possible to 'discover' penicillin at the lower temperatures, complete failure to do so at 72–74°F, as occurred in the experiment I have just quoted, is comparatively unusual. There is frequently some inhibition but not always sufficiently obvious to be detected unless the examiner is actually looking for it. Much also depends on a series of factors that can modify the rate of growth of either the mould or the microbes. If, for example, the mould colony develops quickly because large numbers of recently formed spores are inoculated, penicillin may be formed sufficiently soon to bring about marked and easily recognizable inhibition at as high a temperature as 74–77°F. But a heavy implant of young staphylococci, producing either a confluent sheet of growth or masses of closely adjacent colonies, has the opposite effect, their growth being so rapid that at as low a temperature as 68–72°F there may be only slight or even no inhibition.

Because of these variables it is not possible to state in very precise terms what is the uppermost temperature that will permit the discovery of penicillin following accidental contamination of a culture plate left on the bench without incubation. But in view of the fact that the spores being airborne will be so few in number that unusually rapid growth and production of penicillin is unlikely, and because most culture plates are seeded in such a way that rapid rather than slow growth of the staphylococci is likely to occur, it is improbable that the formation of penicillin is likely to be detected on culture plates kept much above 68°F.

It is not, however, essential that so low a temperature be maintained for very long. All that is required is sufficient time to enable the mould to grow and produce penicillin. At temperatures below 68°F, 4 or 5 days are quite sufficient. Once penicillin is being produced a rise in temperature is of no consequence because lysis occurs as soon as the staphylococci begin to multiply.

If, then, the temperature of the culture plate evidently played so important a part in the discovery of penicillin, we must consider whether that of his laboratory had been low enough while he was away on holiday. Taking 68°F (20°C) for 5 days as the upper limit allowable, he had very little leeway. Most laboratories in this country tend to remain at or above this level for long periods in the year. Even in winter, some kind of artificial heating seldom allows the temperature to fall much below it. Greater fluctuations are probable during the late spring, summer and early autumn when artificial heating may not beemployed if the weather becomes cold. But a temperature of 61–63°F (16·1–17·2°C) is, on the whole, too cold for comfort when sitting at a bench, despite its being suitable for the 'discovery' of penicillin.

Much will, of course, depend on the location of the laboratory. Whether it faces south, how much sun it gets, whether it is, as it were, embedded in a large building, and so on; but even in the absence of artificial heating the temperature will generally be too high.

Fleming's laboratory was, however, somewhat unusual. It was a small room about 10 feet high, 12 feet wide and 10 feet deep. But it was not a rectangle. It was in reality a large bow window on the second floor of a turret on the south-east corner of St Mary's Hospital, projecting into Praed Street. There were, accordingly, three windows in the front: one facing due south and the others south-west and south-east. There was, in addition, a fourth facing due east, which, as can be seen in the photograph has since been bricked up.

It was kept warm enough in the winter by a gas fire, but during the rest of the year its temperature could fluctuate violently for it caught the sun during most of the day, but being well above street level and projecting as it did, it was a a target for cold winds coming from the east and south. It could, accordingly, become very cold when the wind blew.

Assuming that Fleming's culture plate had been seeded with staphylococci and contaminated by the mould at the same time, shortly before he went away for his holiday at the end of July or beginning of August, was the weather at that time such that the

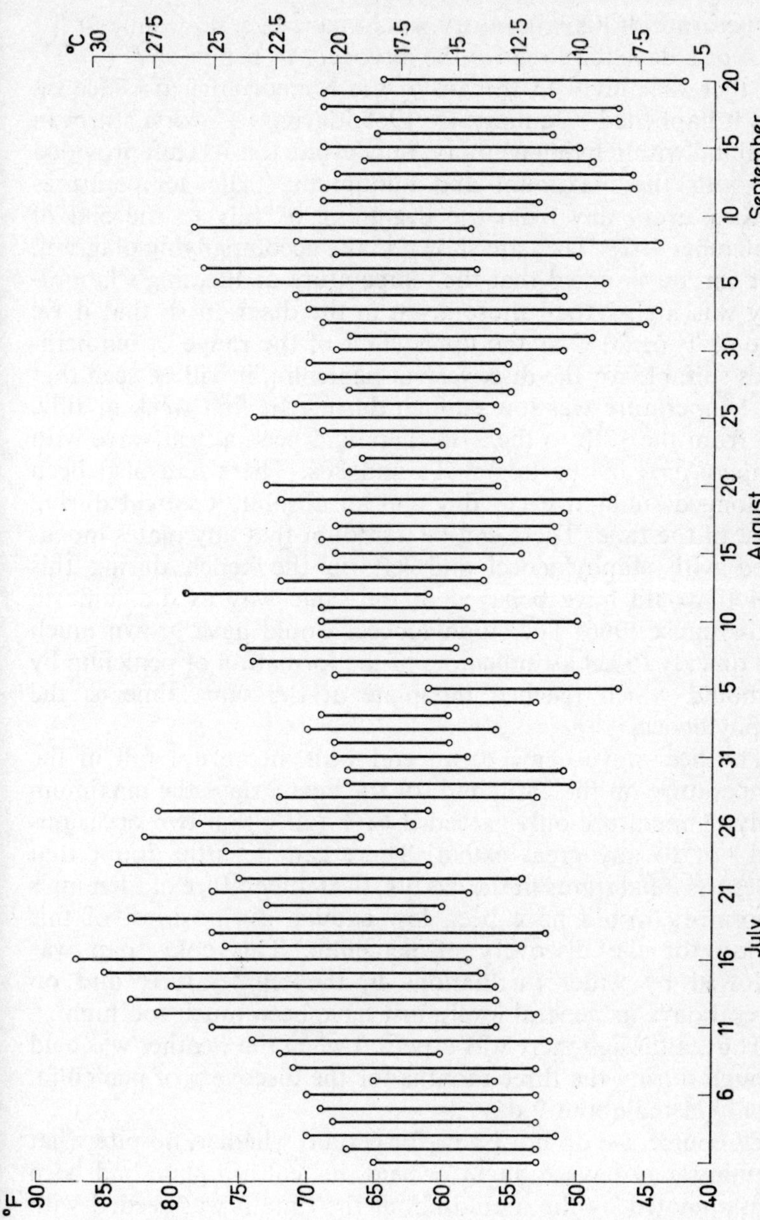

Fig. 1. Daily maximum and minimum temperatures at Kew during July, August and September, 1928.

temperature of his laboratory would have been low enough for the 4 or 5 days required for the discovery of penicillin?

I therefore invoked the aid of the Meteorological Office on – as it happened – January 15, 1968, during the worst storm in Scotland within living memory, but despite this its staff provided me with the maximum and minumum shade temperatures at Kew every day from the beginning of July to the end of September 1928. They are shown in the accompanying diagram.

It can be assumed that the temperature of Fleming's laboratory was higher than those given in the diagram so that if we take 68°F or 20°C as the upper limit of the range of temperatures suitable for the discovery of penicillin, it will be seen that the temperature was low enough during the first week in July, but from the 10th to the 27th there had been a heat-wave with temperatures in the upper 70s and 80s. There had also been prolonged sunlight every day and an absolute drought during most of the time. There can be no doubt that any plates inoculated with staphylococci and left on the bench during this period would have behaved in the same way as did mine in mid-August 1966. The staphylococci would have grown much too quickly to act as indicators of the formation of penicillin by a mould which reached the plate at the same time as the staphylococci.

The heat-wave came to an end with an abrupt fall in the temperature on the 28th, and for the next 9 days the maximum daily temperature only exceeded 68°F (20°C) on two occasions and not to any great extent. There can be little doubt that unless its inhabitants lit the gas fire, the temperature of Fleming's laboratory would have been low enough during most of this period for the discovery of penicillin. This cold snap was followed by wider fluctuations in the temperature, and on several days its general level must have been much too high.

Thus, although there was a period when the weather was cold enough during the three months for the discovery of penicillin, it only lasted about 9 days.

Of course, we do not know for certain whether, despite what Fleming may have thought or said, his culture plate had been contaminated by the mould about the time it was seeded with staphylococci and then left on the bench in a laboratory whose temperature was low enough for the 5 days required, but I have been unable to find any other way to 'discover' penicillin under the conditions in which he was operating.

It is, however, quite possible that this may have been the real history of the culture plate. All he said in his original paper was that it was one of a number that had been 'set aside' in the laboratory. But it must be remembered that the work he was doing was a consequence of his having read the paper by Bigger, Boland and O'Meara to which I have already alluded.[4] In order to produce their variants, they had purposely omitted to incubate their plates and left them on the bench at room temperature, sometimes for as long as 52 days. It is difficult to believe that, at some stage in the proceedings, Fleming did not do the same and this may be what he meant when he said that he had set aside his plates. But there is no mention of his omitting to incubate the plate in the original paper or in the article on the staphylococci in the *System of Bacteriology* he wrote about that time.

It is more probable that the 'setting aside' was another way of describing the hoarding of culture plates to which Fleming was much addicted. It may well be, therefore, that the plate that was responsible for the discovery of penicillin had been seeded shortly before he went away for his holiday, but instead of being put into the incubator had got mixed up with the other plates on his bench that were destined to stay there until his return. The only other possibility is that he merely forgot to incubate it or that the gas went out. But whatever the real explanation may be, the plate cannot have been incubated in the usual way.

All this may perhaps explain why Fleming was, apparently, never able to 're-discover' penicillin. According to Dr Howard Hughes and Dr Lewis Holt who were his close associates for many years, he made many attempts to do so but never succeeded.

If, then, the history of the culture plate had been more or less as I have suggested, the phenomenon on which the discovery of penicillin depended cannot possibly be the comparatively common occurrence so many commentators have assumed it to be. In the first place, it is very unusual for incubation of culture plates to be omitted or even forgotten in any laboratory in which organisms such as staphylococci, streptococci or pneumococci that are susceptible to penicillin, are being studied. Incubation is less common a procedure in laboratories in which organisms from the soil or water are being examined because such organisms generally multiply best at room temperature. But the more susceptible organisms I have mentioned are seldom, if ever, encountered in such laboratories.

In the second place, the fact that the contamination of the plate must occur about the time it is being seeded with staphylococci, reduces very considerably the number of times the phenomenon is likely to be reproduced.

In the third place, the necessity for a comparatively low temperature over a period of about 5 days following the seeding of the plate imposes severe limits on the number of countries and laboratories in which the discovery could be made. No laboratory in a tropical country, for example, would ever be cool enough in the absence of air-conditioning. Those in countries with continental climates such as most of North America, the eastern half of Europe and the whole of northern Asia would be too hot in summer, and central heating in the winter would act in much the same way. Even in countries with temperate climates such as Britain, there are, for reasons I have already discussed, only comparatively short periods in the year when the temperature is likely to be low enough.

Taking all these limitations into consideration, the odds against the occurrence of the phenomenon become almost astronomical. Its rarity becomes even greater when we consider the probable origin of the mould itself. This requires a chapter of its own.

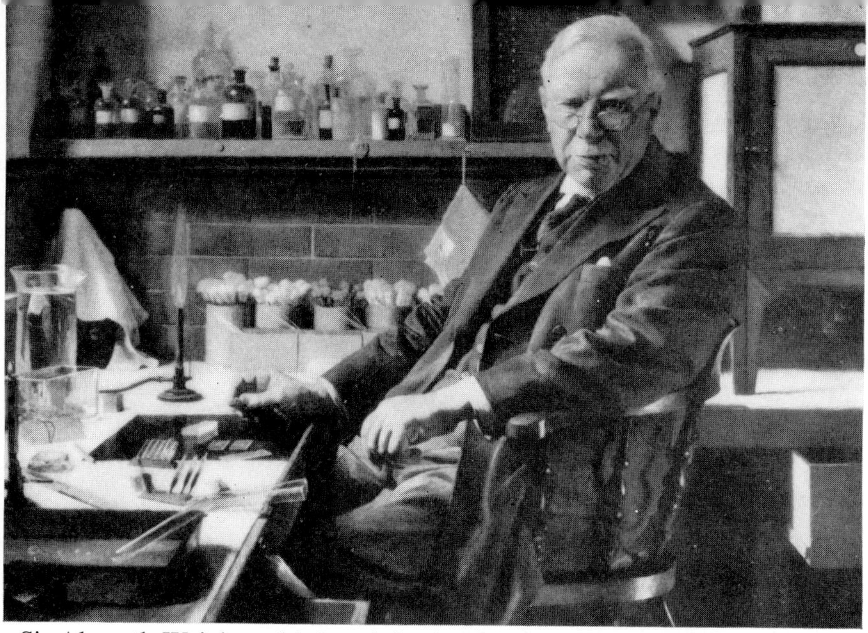

I. Sir Almroth Wright at his bench in the old Inoculation Department soon after the discovery of penicillin. (portrait by Sir Gerald Kelly R.A.).

Staff of the Inoculation Department, St Mary's Hospital, shortly before the discovery of penicillin. *Top row:* L. Colebrook, R. Hare, I. H. Maclean, E. W. Todd, F. Ridley. *Middle row:* A. B. Porteous, R. T. Mummery, J. Matthews, A. E. Wright, A. Fleming, R. M. Fry, A. F. Hayden. *Bottom row:* C. B. Dyson, F. Martley, J. Freeman, C. G. Schoneboom, D. N. E. Thomas.

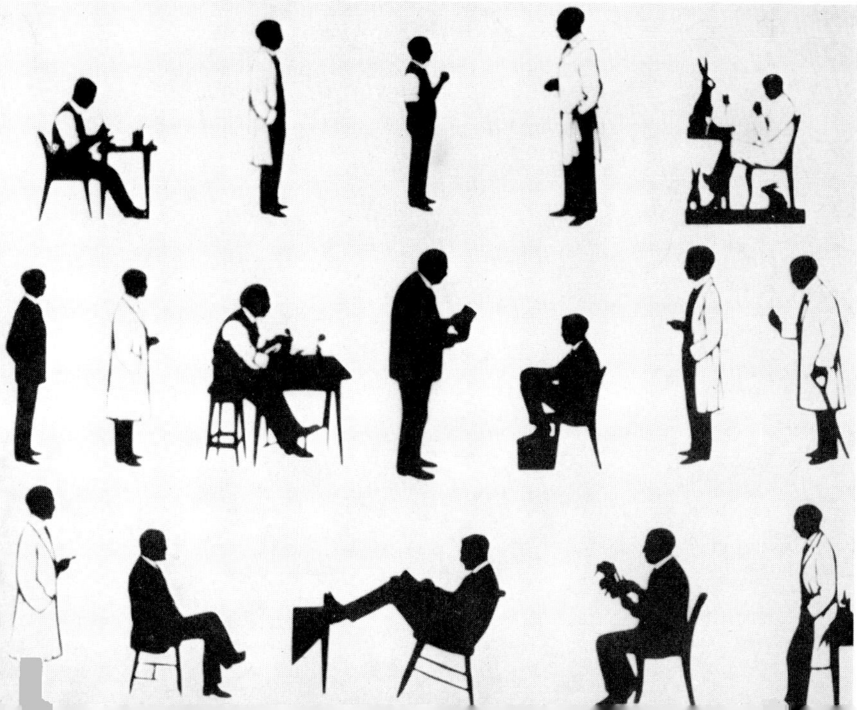

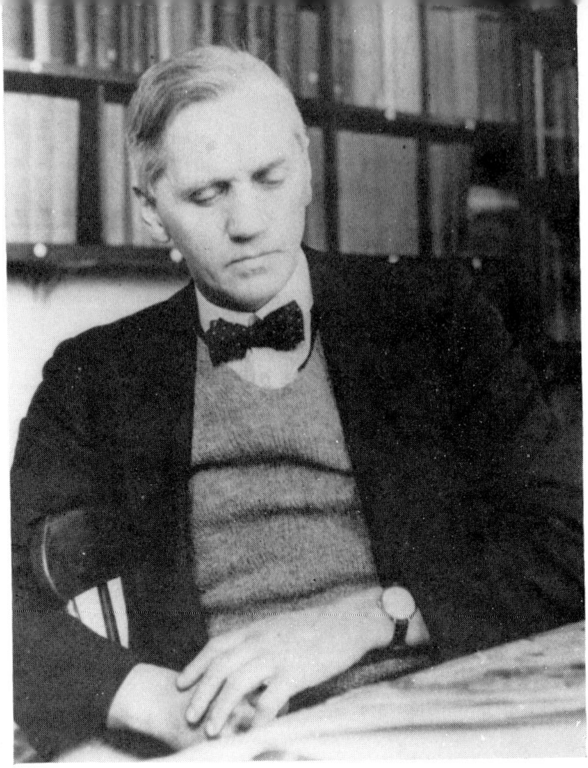

II. Alexander Fleming at the time of the discovery of penicillin.

Fleming's original culture plate showing absence of staphylococcal colonies in the vicinity of the mould.

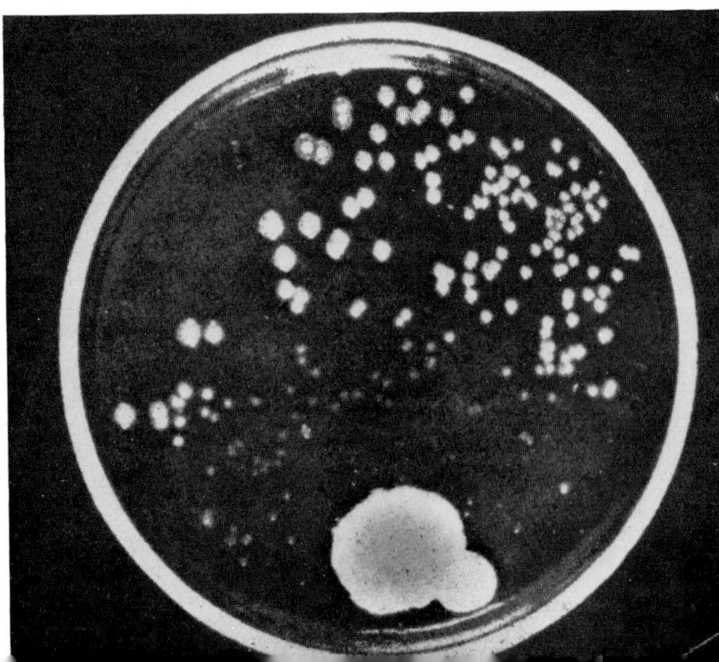

Chapter 4

The Origin of the Mould

The general consensus of opinion as to the origin of the mould spore that alighted on Fleming's culture plate is that it had come from Praed Street, entering his laboratory by way of the window. The Biography, for example, refers to 'the mysterious mould from Praed Street' and, in another place, 'the spore carried by the wind'. Fleming himself seems to have been less certain, for in a speech at the Mayo Clinic he pleaded ignorance, 'a mould spore coming from I don't know where, dropped on the plate',[35] but in his Rectoral Address at Edinburgh he went so far as to say that the 'penicillium had dropped through the window'. There are, however, many reasons for doubting all of this.

In the first place, the window was seldom if ever opened. One powerful reason for this is that the room would have been too noisy. Praed Street is a narrow canyon that so magnifies the roar of the traffic in any room facing on to it that ordinary speech becomes almost inaudible.

Nor do good bacteriologists work on benches immediately beneath an open window, because this is one of the best methods of obtaining contamination of culture plates by unwanted moulds or microbes. And although this may have led to the discovery of penicillin, it is, for all that, thoroughly bad bacteriology. Most bacteriologists, accordingly, keep their windows shut even though it may entail something approaching heat stroke in hot weather.

In any event, for reasons I have made plain, hot weather is not suitable for the discovery of penicillin. It requires an environment that is cool and, if possible, one that is actually cold, 68°F (20°C) being the highest temperature permissible and better still if it is a few degrees lower. Such weather is not likely to tempt anyone to open his window.

Nor would the opening of windows in Fleming's laboratory have been easy. In fact, it would have been something approaching a major operation. Mere words would fail to convey why this should be so. Only by actually seeing the laboratory could the difficulties be appreciated. Nor is there a photograph available that was taken at the time. But fortunately, through the good offices of Dr Howard Hughes, I have been able to obtain prints made by the photographic department of St Mary's Hospital of a reconstruction which Mr P. Flood who had been one of Fleming's technicians, created in the room that had been Fleming's laboratory during the penicillin period. Although there had been an interval of about 25 years, it was a remarkable effort on his part for every detail is accurate. It is an exact replica of the bench at which penicillin was discovered.

All the windows consisted of two panes of glass, and either the upper or the lower could be opened. But it is obvious from the photograph that so small a man as Feming could not have reached even the lower, and still less the upper, while standing on the floor. It would have been difficult for a tall man, so that whoever tried to do it would have had to start by climbing up on to the bench. But the latter was so cluttered that it would have been essential to clear it first. This would not only have been a nuisance, but would have to be repeated to get the window shut before he went home.

If the lower pane was to be opened, nothing whatever could be done until all the boxes of test tubes on the window sill had been removed, because they contained Fleming's store of dangerous microbes which were used for experiments or demonstrations to students. Once the window was open, some of them might have been precipitated on to the heads of passers-by in the street below, with consequences that might have been serious.

Although the window shown in the photograph would have been the most troublesome, the three others would have been little less. Thus, with all this to be gone through, it is perhaps not surprising that Fleming's windows generally remained shut whatever the weather.

If, then, the spore did not get into his laboratory by way of the window, it must have entered by the door. Is there any evidence to support this contention? There is – in fact a great deal which no one seems to have thought of, but which shows that the phenomenon that led to the discovery of penicillin is an even rarer occurrence than anyone has ever imagined it to be.

The events that almost certainly led to the contamination of Fleming's culture plate started months before when Dr Storm van Leeuwen, the distinguished Dutch allergist, came to London and gave a series of lectures at St Thomas's Hospital to which Freeman and I went. Van Leeuwen advanced a theory that some patients suffer from asthma because they are allergic to moulds growing in the foundations and floor boards of their houses. He therefore instituted a method of treatment that involved the patients being removed from the evil influence of moulds by incarcerating them in bungalows, whose sole means of ventilation were tall chimneys sufficiently high to draw air unpolluted by moulds into their interiors. So successful was this method that, in time, these chimneys became a prominent feature of the skyline of Leyden.

Freeman was greatly impressed by the idea that moulds might cause asthma, and persuaded Wright to appoint a young Irish mycologist, C. J. La Touche, to isolate moulds from houses inhabited by suitable asthma patients so that the mould could be identified, and extracts made from it and used for desensitization of the patient. In a very short time La Touche acquired an imposing array of moulds of all kinds. He also grew them in quantity and made the necessary extracts.

As it happens, moulds are more difficult to handle than microbes because, in the course of growth, they produce enormous numbers of spores that are so light that they are easily carried long distances by air currents. Since it is almost impossible to avoid loading the atmosphere with spores, when working with moulds, most mycologists carry out their operations inside fume cupboards or under hoods in order to prevent it. But, as it was one of the inviolable traditions of Wright's laboratory that there must be something wrong about any research that required elaborate apparatus, La Touche had to do the best he could without them. Moreover, the room in which he worked had not been fitted up as a laboratory. He had to use tables instead of benches and do without cupboards or drawers.

This makeshift laboratory was in the same turret in the south-east corner of the building as Fleming's, and immediately below it. Both had doors that opened on to stairs surrounding a lift, and Fleming's was practically always open.

It is therefore a tenable hypothesis that the spore that alighted on Fleming's culture plate had originated in La Touche's laboratory, got into the staircase, and came into his laboratory by way of the door and not the window.

It is, of course, impossible to prove this theory. But confirmation comes from the fact that, soon after the discovery of penicillin, one of Fleming's first tasks was to ascertain whether other species of moulds produced substances with similar properties. He accordingly examined strains identified as *Eidamia viridescens*, *Botrytis cineria*, *Aspergillus fumigatus*, *Sporotrichum* and *Cladosporium*, none of which produced an antibacterial substance similar to penicillin. But he also examined eight strains of *Penicillium.* Of these, only one 'produced any inhibitory substance and that one possessed exactly the same cultural characters as the original one from the contaminated plate'. Like so much that Fleming wrote, it is impossible to make out exactly what he meant, but if he implied that, so far as he could ascertain, the two strains were identical, the coincidence is certainly remarkable.

The coincidence becomes even more remarkable when the particular properties of the mould he found on his culture plate are considered. I have already described how Fleming sub-cultured the mould while Pryce was watching him. He continued to sub-culture it at intervals all through the years that followed. It was this strain that was used by Florey and Chain for the production of penicillin at Oxford. And when, a year or two later, the Americans began a worldwide search for strains capable of producing as much penicillin as possible, Fleming's was found to be one of the three best out of the many strains they examined. It was, therefore, a very unusual strain of the mould.

If, therefore, Fleming meant that the second strain of *Penicillium* produced penicillin in the same quantity as his own strain and resembled it in other respects as well, it is very difficult to believe that, quite by chance, Fleming should have come upon two different strains each having such unique properties. It is impossible to escape the conclusion that the two strains must have come from the same source.

Unfortunately Fleming does not say where he obtained the moulds he had tested. Allison tells me that he isolated one from an old pair of shoes he found in the studio shed at his country house. Whether he himself isolated any others is not known, but the vast majority were given to him by La Touche.[56] It was certainly he who named them. Fleming knew nothing whatever about the identification of moulds. It may therefore be assumed that although La Touche does not know whether or not the second strain of *Penicillium* had come from his collection, it very probably had. We must therefore consider how he had obtained it.

As I have already mentioned, the moulds that La Touche was studying were all derived from dust and floor sweepings collected in houses inhabited by patients with asthma who were being treated by Freeman. Whatever bent Freeman had for research concerned the patients themselves, and not laboratory experiments. It usually involved obtaining their co-operation for some particular purpose. This generally requires a great deal of trouble on the part of the investigator, not to mention a fair measure of intelligence on the part of the patient. All this takes time. He could not spend sufficient time on any one patient in the enormous clinics he held twice a week in the Department. But it was available when he was seeing private patients in his consulting room in Devonshire Place. Within limits he could take as much time as was necessary. It is therefore extremely probable that the research was being conducted with the co-operation of private patients.

Since private patients have to pay fees, it can be concluded that the patient came from a prosperous household. It may well be that the unknown asthmatic whose illness provided the dust that led to the discovery of penicillin came from one of the squares or crescents of Belgravia, Mayfair or Kensington whose tall Victorian houses have basements that are nearly always sufficiently damp to provide an almost ideal environment for the growth of moulds. It is a pity we do not know the address. It would have been a suitable recipient of one of the commemorative blue plaques that add colour to the streets of the Metropolis.

Not long after assisting in the discovery of penicillin, La Touche left the Inoculation Department (and has now become one of the foremost medical mycologists in this country, working in the General Infirmary in Leeds). Before going, he identified the mould. He considered it to be *Penicillium rubrum*. But when it was submitted, some years later, to Dr C. Thom, one of the leading mycologists in North America, he identified it as *Penicillium notatum*. I do not think that this is any reflection on La Touche's abilities because species-differentiation amongst the moulds has always been difficult. Moreover, he was handicapped by an entire absence of literature on moulds in the departmental library, the one book he required was out of print, and the colours reproduced in the only book he possessed were wrong.[56]

Such, then, is what I conceive to be the background to the discovery of penicillin. An accidental observation it is true, but what an accident, depending as it did on a whole series of apparently unrelated events. The choice of Fleming to write a chapter in a book; the publication of a paper in a scientific journal that prompted him to enquire further; lectures by a Dutch physician that led to the appointment of a mycologist; his working in a laboratory directly beneath that of Fleming; his having the good fortune to isolate a powerful penicillin-producing strain of the mould; his having inadequate apparatus so that the atmosphere became loaded with spores; the high probability that Fleming either forgot to incubate his culture plate or purposely omitted to do so; the fact that Fleming's own laboratory was peculiarly sensitive to outside temperatures;

that a cold spell came at a time of the year which is usually unsuitable for the discovery; the visit to Fleming by Pryce that led the former to look again at a plate he had already inspected and discarded; and its having escaped destruction because of entirely inadequate methods for the disposal of used culture plates. All these events, acting in concert, brought to Fleming's notice a phenomenon that cannot, even now, be reproduced unless the conditions in which the experiment is carried out are exactly right. Had only one link in this chain been broken, Fleming would have missed his opportunity.

And if, as Ehrlich used to say, scientific discovery depends partly on *Geld* or money, partly on *Geduld* or patience, partly on *Geschick* or brains and partly on *Glück* or luck, it was the last of them that was almost entirely responsible for the discovery of penicillin. It was, surely, the supreme example in all scientific history, of the part that luck may play in the advancement of knowledge.

Chapter 5

Variations on a Chemical Theme

Following its discovery, Fleming studied penicillin in considerable detail. He found that, when added to the ordinary digest broth of the laboratory, the mould grew in the form of a thick wrinkled felt floating on the surface. The broth below, when freed from the mould by filtration, would prevent growth of staphylococci and other organisms in quite high dilution. It was obviously something derived from the mould that had produced the phenomenon he had seen on his culture plate.

In accordance with standard departmental practice, broth which had acquired this new property was promptly given a nickname, 'mould juice'. Not until later was the active principle called penicillin, derived from *Penicillium*, the generic name for the mould that produces it. The name was first used in the original paper published in 1929, but Fleming does not mention who was responsible for it. I had always assumed that Wright was the real author if only because one of his hobbies was the invention of new words. They were almost always derived from the Greek, and in his later papers he generally began with a long dissertation on nomenclature. It is not, therefore, very surprising that (so V. D. Allison tells me) it was Wright who suggested lysozyme for the ferment in tears that Fleming discovered. But Allison also tells me that Fleming himself was the author of penicillin. I do not know what Wright's reaction was, but he would not have been human had he not been furious when he eventually realized that the most important of the many new terms that emanated from his laboratory had been invented by someone else; and what was worse, someone who knew no Greek.

The paper describing the discovery of penicillin and the investigations that followed was sent to the *British Journal of Experimental Pathology* on May 10, 1929. It was published in the June issue of that Journal. In it may be found an account of all the main properties of penicillin. Many of them do not concern the use of penicillin for treatment, for which reason they need not be referred to here. But four properties suggested that it might have value for this purpose; that it could kill several species of disease-producing organisms; that it could do so when diluted quite considerably; that it was, apparently, harmless; and that it was readily diffusible.[24]

To ascertain what species of microbes were susceptible, Fleming used the now familiar ditch plate, originally invented by him for the study of lysozyme. To prepare such a plate he took an ordinary agar culture plate and with a scalpel cut a hole, trough or gutter in the agar. Into this cavity, melted agar containing mould juice was poured. When it had set, cultures of different species of organisms were streaked across both the ditch and the rest of the plate. It was then incubated and those species that were susceptible failed to grow on the agar of the ditch but did so on the rest of the streak.

In this way, it was determined that a whole series of disease-producing organisms were sensitive. The most important were streptococci, pneumococci, gonococci and meningococci. Most of the bacilli such as those causing typhoid and dysentery were insusceptible.

To measure the efficiency of penicillin, he used mould juice after 5 days' growth of the mould. A series of dilutions were made in broth, to each of which was added a suspension of staphylococci. The tubes were then incubated overnight, and growth of the organisms was inhibited in the tubes containing most penicillin. The highest dilution in which this occurred was recorded as the end point, or 'titre', as it is generally called.

It was found that a good sample of mould juice could be diluted 600 or 800 times before it ceased to prevent growth of the organisms; but 200 or 300 times was more usual. Thus, the penicillin in crude mould juice was a comparatively powerful antibacterial substance, considerably more powerful than carbolic acid – which cannot be diluted more than 200 times – about the same as the cresols such as lysol, but much weaker than some other antiseptics such as the flavines that can be diluted as much as 4,000 times before they cease to act.

Tests to ascertain whether the penicillin in mould juice was harmful were carried out in a variety of ways. In preliminary experiments it was administered by mouth, or as Craddock told me; 'I grew the mould in milk and the resulting substance was very much like Stilton cheese and I ate it with no ill effects. Eventually a man was admitted to the ward and he was given the stuff three times a day by mouth. It did him no harm.'

Further tests, described somewhat laconically in the original paper, were also carried out as follows: 'Constant irrigation of large infected surfaces in man was not accompanied by any toxic symptoms, while irrigation of the human conjunctiva had no irritant effect.' 'Twenty cc. injected intravenously into a rabbit were not more toxic than the same quanity of broth.' 'Half a cc. injected intraperitoneally into a mouse weighing about 20 gm. induced no toxic symptoms.' '*In vitro* penicillin which completely inhibits the growth of staphylococci in a dilution of 1 in 600 does not interfere with leucocytic function more than ordinary broth.'

The fourth attribute that recommended penicillin to Fleming was that it was more diffusible than other antibacterial substances. When incorporated into agar, it spread centrifugally to a much greater distance. This would give it great advantages when used for the local treatment of an infected wound for example.

Substances with all these four properties are common enough nowadays. Several hundred must be known and more are being found every year. But in 1928 it was a very different matter. They could be numbered on the fingers of one hand. So obviously unique was penicillin that its chemotherapeutic potentialities would have to be examined very carefully.

Many obstacles would have to be overcome before it could be

tested. One of the first was to decide how it was to be used. Chemotherapeutic agents must come into contact with the microbes before they can act on them. But this can be brought about in two entirely different ways.

If the microbes are accessible from the outside, that is, when they are infecting the skin or mucous membranes such as those of the eye, nose, throat, mouth, vagina or urethra, or when they are causing infection of open shallow wounds such as burns, ulcers and the like, the agent can be directly applied in an irrigating fluid, in a powder or in a paste.

Alternatively, the agent can be transported to the microbes by the blood stream from an injection site or, if it has been swallowed, from the alimentary canal. The surface infections I have enumerated above can, or course, be treated in this way. But, and this is the important point, it is the only method by which the agent can be brought to the scene of action when the organisms are causing a deep-seated infection such as meningitis, pneumonia, osteomyelitis or puerperal fever.

Of the two routes by which the substance can reach the infecting organisms, direct application from the outside is by far the easiest. Within limits, the agent need not be completely devoid of toxicity, the presence of other substances in the fluid need not matter, and no great quantity may be necessary. There is no doubt whatever that Fleming thought that even crude mould juice could be used in this way.

The second method of treatment in which the drug is carried to the infected area by the blood stream is an entirely different proposition. In the first place, the whole body must be saturated, as it were, so that an effective concentration can be brought to bear at the site of infection. This is by no means easy to achieve, largely because the body contains about 15 litres of blood and nearly the same amount of other fluids as well. Preliminary calculations showed that even though crude mould juice can be diluted several hundred times before ceasing to act, large volumes would be required to provide only one dose; probably 1 or even 2 litres. And since penicillin in the blood stream would be excreted by the kidneys, further doses would have to be given. So large a volume of fluid administered repeatedly could not possibly be tolerated. Thus whatever else was done, a great deal of the water would have to be removed.

In the second place, it was generally assumed in the 1920s that any agent would have to be administered by intravenous injection. But this could be dangerous if other substances besides penicillin were also present. In this respect, mould juice was one of the worst fluids that could be imagined. It was, basically, broth made by the tryptic digestion of condemned meat or the heart of a bullock. Although it had been found by that time that moulds will grow in simpler synthetic media of less dangerous composition, I doubt whether Fleming would have known this. But he did know that the intravenous injection of protein solutions could produce serious symptoms known as protein shock in which the patient becomes restless, his temperature rises, and within an hour or so he has a series of severe rigors. These ultimately cease, the temperature falls and the patient recovers. Drastic measures of this nature were actually employed for the treatment of rheumatoid arthritis and were sufficiently successful for the patients to ask for more. But they might have killed a patient with a sufficiently severe infection to require the use of penicillin. Whatever else was done, therefore, the proteins, as well as any other toxic substances the mould might have produced, would have to be removed.

The third requirement was that the penicillin must be sufficiently stable to enable supplies to be prepared beforehand, ready for the treatment of patients as soon as they reached hospital. It was quite out of the question to put off the production of penicillin until the patient became ill. Perhaps this was the most important of these requirements.

The purification, concentration and stabilization of penicillin was a chemical problem. Here Fleming was seriously handicapped. He was no chemist, and what little he knew can have been no more than the remnants of what he had learned as a student many years before. What is more, organic chemistry and biochemistry, which were the main requirements for the problem, were both probably closed books to him.

There was no chemist on the staff of the Inoculation Department. Dr Roche Lynch, who was the chemical pathologist to the hospital, had had chemical training. But he was one of the forensic specialists retained by the Home Office, and spent most of his time looking for arsenic in the bodies of murder victims and attending the trials of the suspected murderers. With this preoccupation he had no time to devote to an unstable substance derived from a mould.

Fortunately, however, Frederick Ridley, a young ophthalmologist, was at that time working with Fleming on the lysozyme in tears. He had had rather more chemical training than most of us because he had had to take the biochemistry course for B.Sc. students at Birmingham University, where he was studying, in order to prepare himself for the M.B. and B.S. degree examinations of London University. This background automatically qualified him to take charge of the chemical investigation of penicillin.

Stuart Craddock was also called upon to help. His job was to provide the raw material for Ridley, but he also carried out a great many of the titrations. Both of them worked hard and made many significant advances, most of which were neither published nor referred to by Fleming. I propose to describe them in some detail, and in this I have been greatly helped by both Ridley and Craddock.

The first objective was to obtain mould juice with as high a concentration of penicillin as possible. The mould was inoculated into broth in '150–200c.c. flasks or flat-sided bottles lying on their side with a wool plug and tin placed over it'. Little penicillin was produced at 37°C (98°F) but 'a large black incubator with a glass door was found and this was kept at about 20°C (68°F). The quality improved greatly and would inhibit staphylococci and streptococci at dilutions up to 1/600 or 1/800'. Many attempts were made to obtain a more satisfactory medium, but in the end they found that 'the digest broth from bullock's heart was the best'.

The bottles and flasks were incubated for about 5 days, when the broth was filtered through an old-fashioned Seitz filter in which the fluid is forced through an asbestos pad from a reservoir holding only 50 c.c. by air pressure produced by a bicycle pump and maintained by a tyre valve.

The next step was to concentrate and, if possible, purify the penicillin in mould juice. Being the first to attempt this, Ridley had nothing to guide him. The one thing he did know was that a great deal of the water would have to be removed and that most of the unwanted substances were proteins. If the penicillin could survive such an ordeal, this alone would be a major step forward.

Ridley's first step was, accordingly, the removal of the water. For this purpose he used vacuum distillation at a low temperature; that is to say, the mould juice was placed in a flask and the air evacuated while the fluid was warmed to a temperature of about 40°C. Under such conditions the fluid boils and the steam is carried away in the vacuum line. Practically all the water and any other volatile substances can be removed in this way.

Although this sounds easy, a great many difficulties were encountered. A satisfactory vacuum was, for example, impossible to obtain when using the water pumps in the laboratory. Being on the second floor the water pressure was insufficient. But Ridley found that a tap in a corridor next to Wright's laboratory was evidently connected to the rising main, because a pump attached to it was much more efficient. Unfortunately it was over a large sink and the only place on which to put their apparatus was the draining slab. Gas for heating had to be brought in by a long tube from the laboratory next door. If these impediments were not enough, the sink itself was in a draughty passage 11 feet long and only 4 feet wide. Below it and projecting here and there was an enormous centrifuge which, fortunately, was seldom used.

Even when carried out under ideal conditions, vacuum distillation is a tricky business. Frothing is liable to occur so that much of the fluid may be lost up the vacuum line. Overheating too – particularly when gas must be used – is an ever present danger. To make matters worse, the distillations generally took a whole day and someone had to be on watch all the time.

The process was further complicated by the discovery that the pH of the fluid was of considerable importance. The symbol pH is scientific shorthand giving in numerical terms the acidity or alkalinity of a solution. The dividing line between the two – when the solution is neutral in reaction – is expressed as 7·0. When the solution is alkaline the pH is greater than 7·0 and when it is acid it is less than 7·0.

The modern electrical methods for the measurement of the pH not being available, they added indicators to samples of the fluid and compared the colours produced with those on colour charts. These showed that, when harvested, the mould juice was markedly alkaline, its pH being 8·5–9·0. If the distillation was attempted, the penicillin rapidly disappeared. But if the pH was brought down to 6·5 or even lower, by adding hydrochloric acid, the penicillin would survive the distillation. Unfortunately the pH tended to rise to dangerous levels as the distillation proceeded. For this reason at intervals of about an hour the vacuum had to be shut off, the flask opened, a sample of fluid withdrawn, its pH determined, acid added and the pH checked. again before the vacuum could be started and the distillation continued.

To complicate matters still more, they suspected towards the end of their investigations that oxygen in the flask might inactivate the penicillin every time they opened it to correct the pH. They therefore filled the flask with hydrogen from a Kipps apparatus whenever they did this. And anyone who has used this apparatus will know how temperamental it can be.

Despite these difficulties, it was possible to remove nearly all the water in this way. And, probably much to their astonishment, very little of the penicillin was lost in the process. This is admirably demonstrated in the protocols of experiments Craddock gave me. Thus, on March 20, they used mould juice whose penicillin titre was 1/100 and a sample of 200 c.c. was evaporated to dryness. To this was added 5 c.c. of distilled water. The titre of this solution was 1/3,000. Corrected for the forty-times concentration, this works out at 1/75, so that allowing for experimental error very little of the penicillin can have disappeared during the evaporation.

Having concentrated the broth in this way, it was now necessary to remove as much of the unwanted proteins as possible.

Alcohol was chosen for this purpose and 45 c.c. of 90 per cent alcohol was added to the 5 c.c. of watery solution obtained in the experiment quoted above. A precipitate formed which was allowed to settle. The titre of the supernatent mixture of alcohol and water was then determined. It was found to be 1/500. Since the concentration was now four times that of the original fluid, this corresponds to a titre of 1/125 in the broth. Thus, very little of the penicillin can have disappeared during these procedures.

In another experiment carried out on April 10, 1,200 c.c. of mould juice with a titre of 1/300 was concentrated to 50 c.c. and 70 c.c. of alcohol added. The precipitated proteins were removed by centrifugation. The titre of the supernatant mixture of alcohol and water was 1/3,000. Since the concentration was ten times, this means that the whole of the penicillin had gone into solution in the alcohol.

These experiments were a major step forward because they showed that penicillin could not be a protein. But of equal importance, they also showed that penicillin was evidently soluble in an organic solvent, and for this reason its molecule could not be very large or complicated.

However valuable these experiments may have been, the fact remains that a solution of penicillin in very nearly pure alcohol is unsuitable for biological tests of any kind. It would have to be in watery solution if it was to be of any use. Ridley solved, or partially solved, this problem by a simple expedient. He removed the alcohol by evaporation, using a vacuum. Or, in his own words; 'We had obtained an absolute alcohol extract which we evaporated to a small syrupy residue not exceeding half a cc in volume. This was redissolved in 5 cc of water and still had a titre of 3,000 or 5,000.' From this it follows that the titre of the syrup must have been about 1/30,000 or 1/50,000. Ridley had therefore not only obtained a considerable amount of concentration but had removed most of the proteins as well. What is more, the titres of these concentrates remained high for a week or 10 days, even when kept liquid in the primitive ice box in the laboratory.

When ether or chloroform were employed instead of alcohol,

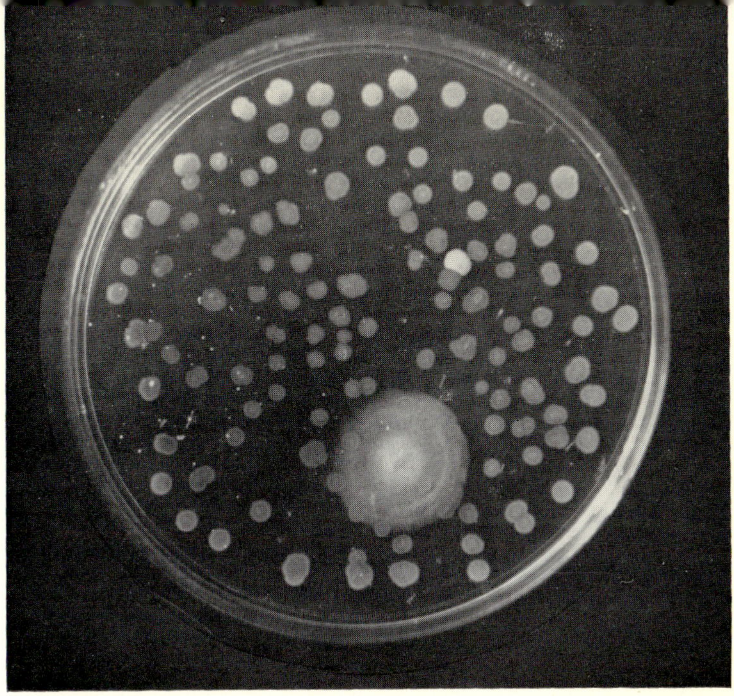

III. Absence of all signs of penicillin activity on a plate contaminated by the mould after the staphylococcal colonies had developed fully.

Inhibition of staphylococcal growth on a plate contaminated by the mould at the time it was seeded with staphylococci and then left on the bench.

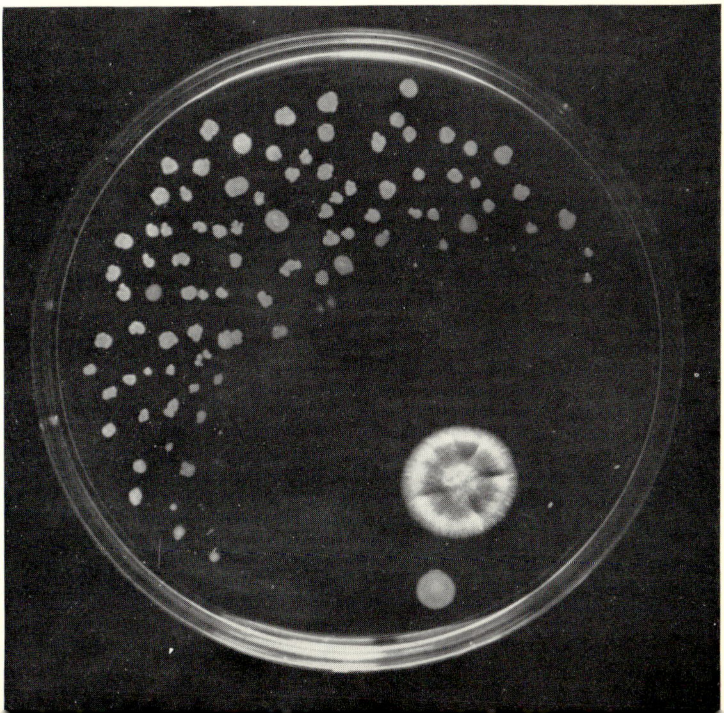

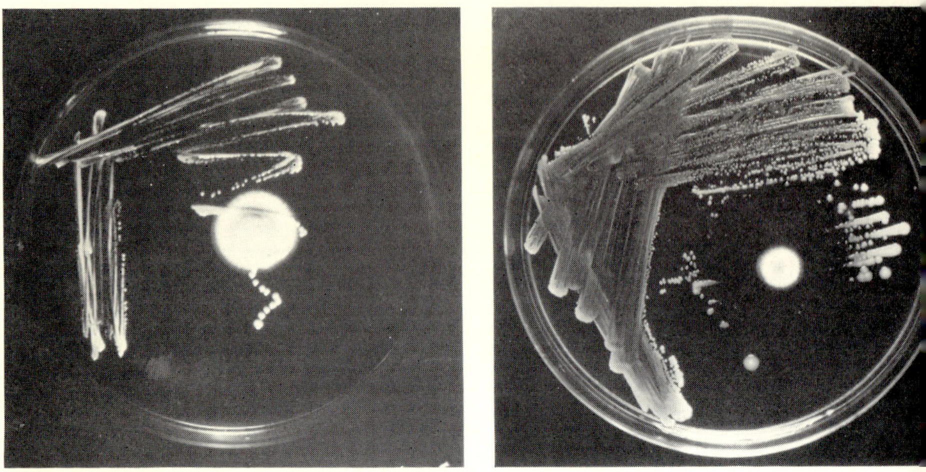

IV. The part that
perature playe
the discovery of
icillin. Both p
were contamin
by the mould at
time they
seeded with sta
lococci but tha
the left was su
quently kept at
74°F and that
the right at
63°F.

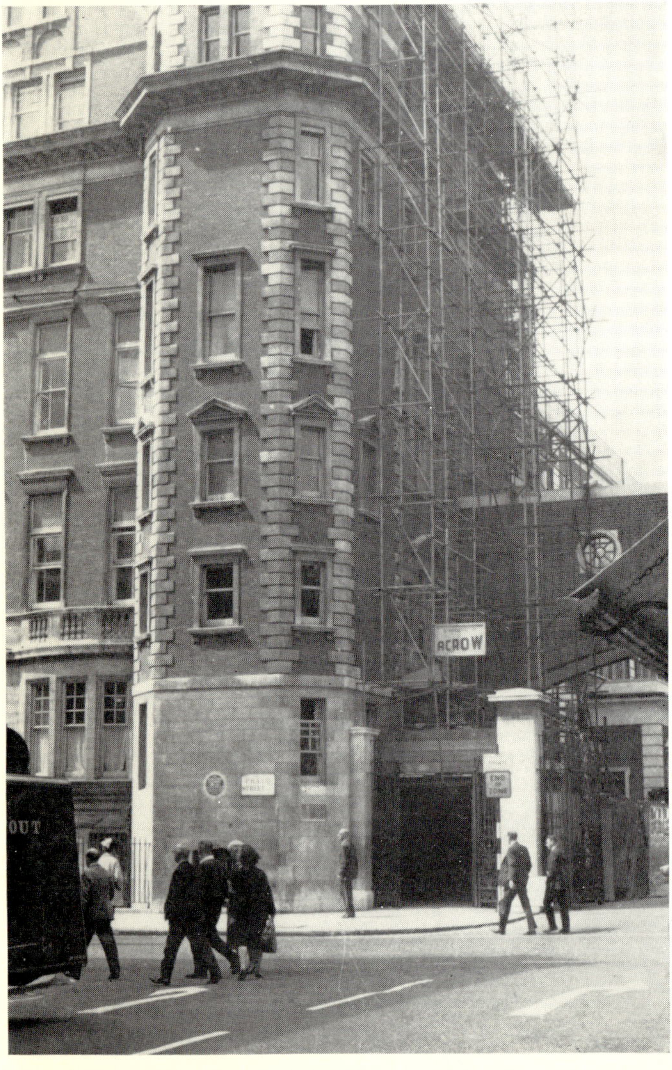

Turret at the so
eastern corner
St Mary's Hos
in which penic
was discove
Ground fl
Secretary's o
First floor:
Touche's lab
tory. Second fl
Fleming's lab
tory. Third fl
Library.

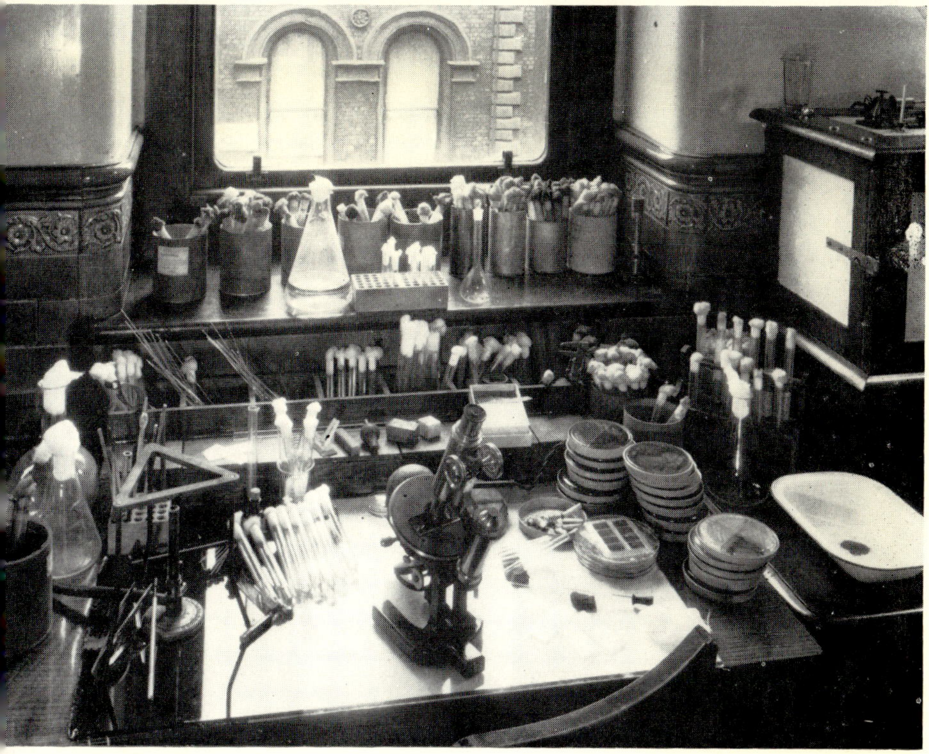

Reconstruction of Fleming's work bench in the room in which penicillin was discovered.

Left: Frederick Ridley. *Right:* S. R. Craddock. Both photographs were taken about the time that penicillin was discovered.

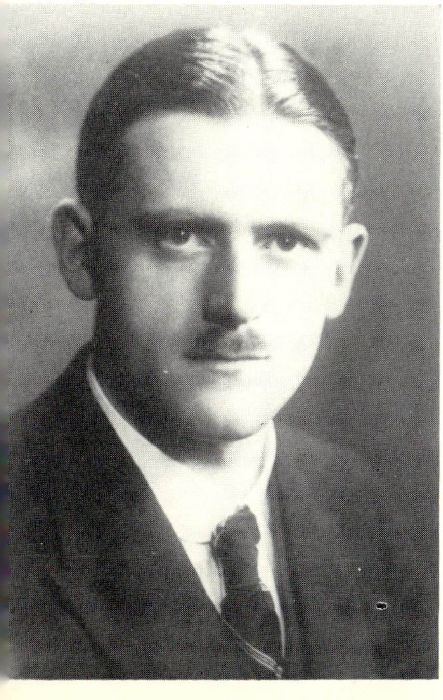

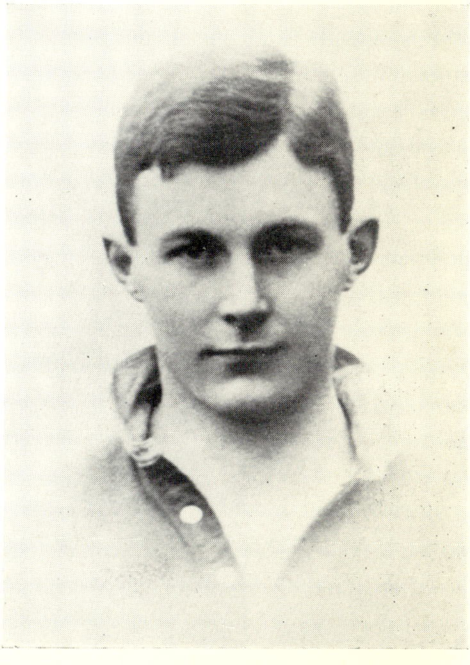

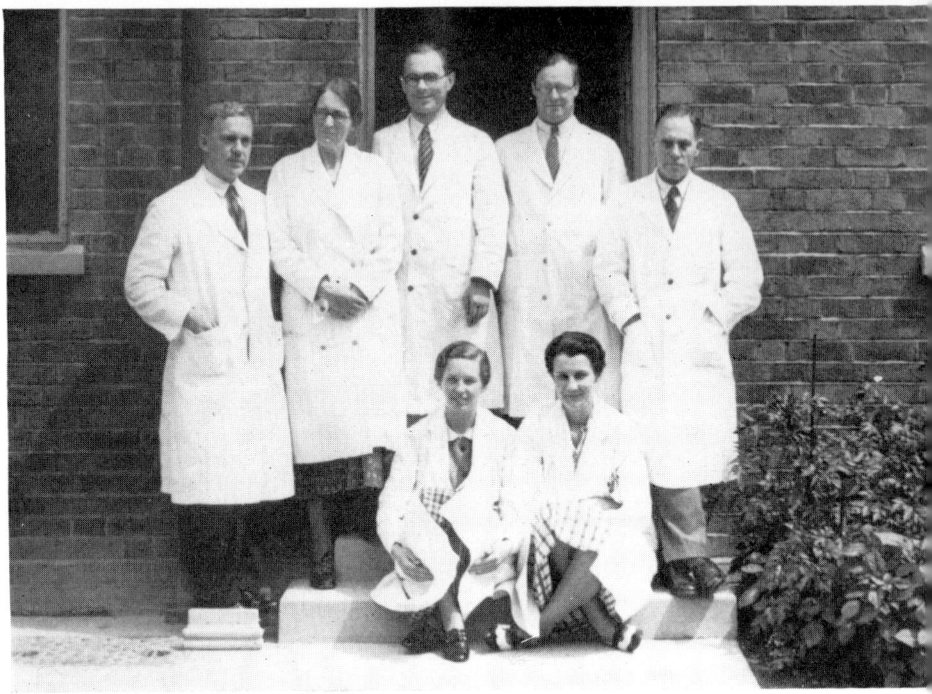

VI. Staff of the laboratories at Q
Charlotte's Hospital, 1931–6.
row, left to right: R. M. Fry, I
Colebrook, A. T. Fuller, R. H
L. Colebrook. *Front row:* Eliza
White, Meave Kenny.

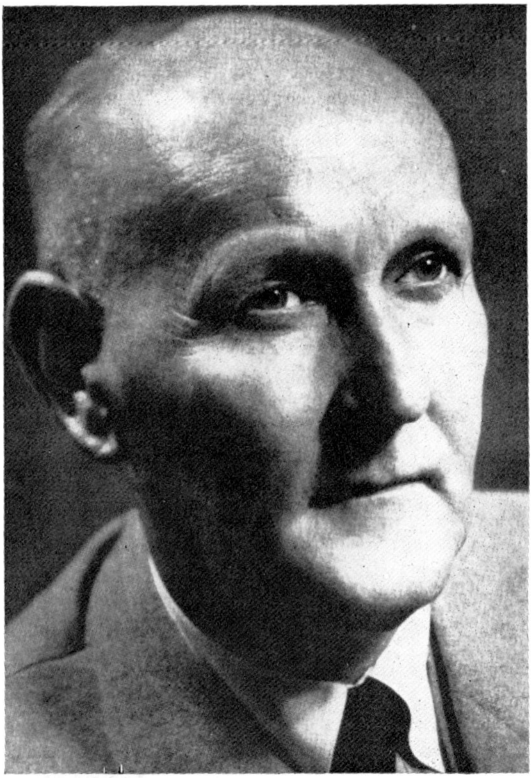

Gerhard Domagk.

no penicillin could be detected in the solvent. But acetone was of some value. Indeed, this discovery was made before it was found that penicillin was soluble in alcohol. Thus, on March 12, a specimen of mould juice whose titre was 1/200 was concentrated to a thick fluid. To this, 4 volumes of acetone were added and the mixture centrifuged. The titre of the supernatant fluid was 1/200 whereas that of the deposit was only 1/20. Acetone itself, tested under the same conditions, had no action on the test organisms.

Acetone was obviously a less efficient solvent than alcohol but the fact remains that it had evidently dissolved an appreciable amount of the penicillin. This was also a discovery of considerable importance.

Ridley also found that acetone could be used for further purification of the high titre concentrates he had obtained by alcoholic extraction. Addition of 2 volumes of acetone brought down a precipitate containing very little penicillin. The precipitate that was produced in this way was found, however, to contain large amounts of the substance that gave both the crude filtrate and concentrates their yellow colour. This meant, in turn, that the colouring matter we now know as crysogenin was not penicillin.

These investigations had provided Fleming with a method for the partial purification of penicillin which, when things went well, gave him all the penicillin in one-tenth or even one-hundredth of the volume of the original broth. Or, as Ridley himself put it, 'By continually adjusting the acidity to pH 6·5 during low temperature (40°C) vacuum distillation, followed by extraction with alcohol and precipitation of an inactive fraction from the alcoholic solution by two volumes of acetone, this gave us a full yield of high potency penicillin. We lost little in the process.'[70]

To most bacteriologists the next step would have been obvious; to ascertain whether these preparations had any value as chemotherapeutic agents. Although only small quantities were available they might have sufficed for mice; and even if they were toxic they need not have been actually lethal.

For technical reasons, such tests could not have been carried out with staphylococci. Streptococci or pneumococci would have been more suitable and small numbers of these organisms generally kill mice within 48 hours. Even if only some of the animals were saved following administration of the concentrates, it would have been a major step forward. But Ridley and Craddock who would have had to provide the material have never heard of any such attempts being made.

Even more remarkable, in my opinion, is the fact that the work was allowed to stop when this stage was reached. This was, partly at least, due to the fact that Ridley left. He had never intended to make bacteriology his career, Ophthalmology was his ambition, and as he was now 27 it was time he started in earnest. (In this he was extremely successful, becoming a member of the staff of Moorfield's Eye Hospital and one of the foremost authorities in the world on contact lenses.) There had been no quarrel or rift but Fleming made no attempt whatever to persuade him to postpone his departure at what would, to most people, have seemed an extremely awkward moment.

Nevertheless, his resignation need not have caused a complete cessation of all activity. Craddock, despite his inexperience, was technically extremely competent and knew enough about the method to have carried on by himself. Moreover, Fleming himself was only 48 years old and certainly not too old to have learned enough chemistry to have helped him in case of need.

It is of course possible that Fleming was not fully aware of all that had been achieved. There is some justification for this because Ridley and Craddock had been working some distance from him in a big laboratory up some stairs and along a corridor. And certainly, there is a remarkable series of omissions in the account he gave in the original paper. It is a single paragraph that reads as follows:

> *Solubility.*—It is freely soluble in water and weak saline solutions. My colleague, Mr Ridley, has found that if penicillin is evaporated at a low temperature to a sticky mass the active principle can be completely extracted by absolute alcohol. It is insoluble in ether or chloroform.

This does, it is true, give the facts or, more correctly, some of them. Quite apart from omitting all mention of the solubility of penicillin in acetone, he says virtually nothing about the procedures employed so that there is no mention of the necessity for a vacuum, the temperature employed is not given, there is no reference to the importance of the pH and that it had to be periodically adjusted to keep it low, there is no indication of the titres of the penicillin in the masses, or whether a watery solution could be obtained from the alcoholic extracts.

A second reason for suspecting that he knew very little about the work is that he never referred to it in after years in papers, lectures or even in private conversations. In fact, he seems to have forgotten all about it.

I therefore asked Craddock whether Fleming had, in fact, been kept fully informed and appreciated what he and Ridley had been doing. In reply, he told me that 'he was "in" on all we did, but I don't think you can say that he directed us in our attempts to concentrate and extract. He tried to help us, but he was as ignorant as we were and we probably read up the various methods of extracting substances more than he did, and we certainly tried them without his help.' Fleming seems to have been equally well informed about the remaining procedures for, to quote Craddock again, 'All the titrations etc. were done by me on his instructions. Each day's work was put on a piece of loose leaf paper and left with him.' He then goes on to say, 'I must make it clear that in all the work I did Flem was behind it all, and this must be quite obvious to anyone who cares to recall that as soon as I started to do any bacteriology, I was channelled into working on his mould juice and was completely inexperienced.'

If, then, Fleming was really conversant with all that had been going on, the only possible conclusion that can be reached to account for its cessation is that by the spring of 1929 he was losing interest in penicillin as a chemotherapeutic substance for the treatment of deep-seated infections. It was primarily for the treatment of this type of infection that the work had started at all. Why, therefore, continue with it if the value of penicillin began to be doubtful?

Craddock too left about a year later, after having helped

Fleming to perfect the technique in which penicillin is used for the isolation of penicillin-insensitive microbes from mixed cultures. Far from Fleming making any attempt to keep him, he encouraged and helped him to obtain an appointment in the Wellcome Research Laboratories at Beckenham. He gave up bacteriology in 1932 and became a general practitioner at Holsworthy in Devon. He remained in close touch with Fleming until the latter died. He had him to stay with him on several occasions, and was in fact one of his closest friends.

In any event, it was about this time that Prof. Harold Raistrick at the London School of Hygiene and Tropical Medicine became interested in penicillin, mostly because it was a product of the growth of a member of the *Penicillium chrysogenum* series of moulds. He had studied the biochemistry of micro-organisms for years and was not only one of the leading authorities in the world on the subject but, as head of the Department of Biochemistry, had ample resources at his disposal.

Because of this it was quite impossible for him to ignore penicillin and he asked Dr P. W. Clutterbuck, one of his assistants, to carry out what is described in their paper as 'the preliminary attempts at isolation of penicillin using Fleming's culture'.[6] The determinations of the titres of penicillin in their preparations required a bacteriological technique and this part of the work was done by Dr (now Prof.) Reginald Lovell, a member of the Department of Bacteriology in the same School. Assistance was also afforded by a mycologist, Mr J. H. V. Charles who was, unfortunately, killed in a road accident shortly after the work had ceased. Except for occasional consultations Raistrick himself took no active part in the investigations.

The paper describing their work was published in 1932 in the *Biochemical Journal*, the authors being given as P. W. Clutterbuck, R. Lovell and H. Raistrick.[6] Only three pages concern penicillin, one being taken up with details of the method used for its titration, about three-quarters of another for the yield and keeping qualities, and the remainder for its chemical behaviour.

Their results may be summarized as follows. The completely

synthetic Czapek Dox medium could be employed for its production instead of digest broth, the main disadvantage being the long time, (16–20 days) required instead of only 5 in the broth. They were also the first to publish a clear statement about the keeping qualities of penicillin. At 0°C, for example, a filtrate of a culture in Czapek Dox medium which would inhibit growth of the pneumococcus at a dilution of 1/1280, was still sufficiently potent to do so at a dilution of 1/320 after 16 weeks. They also found, as indeed had Ridley and Craddock, that by adjusting the pH to 5–6, the penicillin was much more stable than at the original pH of 8–9. Such an adjusted filtrate might remain unchanged for as long as 3 months.

Their third contribution was that by careful acidification of the filtrate with sulphuric acid, to bring down the pH to 3·6, a flocculent yellow precipitate was obtained, containing little penicillin but an appreciable amount of protein and crysogenin, the colouring matter produced by the mould. This alone effected a considerable amount of purification.

It was also found that if the crude filtrate was concentrated by vacuum distillation, the penicillin in the resulting mass would go into solution in still another organic solvent, ether. Whether or not it did so depended on the pH. At 7·2 only a small proportion was taken up, whereas virtually all of it went into solution at pH 2·0. Recovery of the penicillin from the ethereal solution proved to be more difficult. If it was mixed with water and the ether removed by evaporation *in vacuo* at 40–45°C, some of the penicillin could be recovered from the water remaining in the vessel. But there were heavy losses in the process. But, worse still, if the ether was removed by the simple expedient of allowing it to evaporate, there was no penicillin in the residue that remained.

The work seems to have ceased at this point and it is only too obvious that although much was learned about the properties of penicillin, they had got no nearer to the evolution of a method for its purification and concentration than did Ridley and Craddock. It may well be asked why they stopped when they did.

In the first place it is not at all certain that this is what they set out to do. Prof. Lovell doubts whether Fleming approached Raistrick with a request to provide him with a product fit for the treatment of infections. He did not know Raistrick at that time. There is even doubt whether Fleming got so far as to discuss the matter at all, and certainly Lovell had never heard about Ridley's work until I told him in 1965, 37 years after the event. In fact, the only contact seems to have been that Fleming gave them a culture of his mould and had several telephone conversations with Lovell.

In the second place, Raistrick had to investigate penicillin as part of his study of the biochemistry of moulds. Whether Fleming asked him or not, this was part of his job. But he and Clutterbuck were chemists, primarily interested in the products produced by moulds that could be isolated by the ordinary chemical processes, purified and if possible crystallized. Products which disappeared when the ether in which they were dissolved was allowed to evaporate were another matter. To have re-oriented their thinking and their techniques to deal with such a substance would have been a major operation.

Up to this point, the story seems to me perfectly straightforward. Raistrick and his colleagues had looked at the substance because they had to, found that it behaved in so highly abnormal a manner that they were not prepared to spend time and trouble on it, and passed on to other things.

When, however, penicillin was found to be so valuable, Fleming took it upon himself to complicate the matter very badly. In the first place, he used such expressions as, 'even skilled chemists had failed in their attempts to concentrate, stabilize and purify penicillin.'[2] This theme was repeated in a number of obituaries such as that in the *Journal of Pathology and Bacteriology*, 'the failure of Raistrick and his team to isolate the active principle',[17] and in the Obituary Notices of Fellows of the Royal Society, 'Raistrick and his colleagues had failed to extract and purify the active principle'.[11]

In the second place, he stated on more than one occasion that this was the fault of the bacteriologists. Thus, in a lecture in America, 'the bacteriologists in the institution did not fully co-operate',[35] and twice in the Harben Lectures, 'lack of bacteriological co-operation hindered their work', and 'Raistrick lacked complete bacteriological co-operation'.[34]

It is very doubtful whether any of this is true. For reasons I have already given, it is improbable that Raistrick was ever asked to find a method for the purification of penicillin. Fleming may have hoped that he would. But that is a different matter. Nor is it likely that the work came to an end because the bacteriologists failed to help. Lovell has told me that he remained at the School of Hygiene until the autumn of 1933, a full year after the publication of the paper. There had been no quarrel or rift with Clutterbuck with whom he had worked amicably, and Prof. Topley, his chief, allowed him a free hand to do as he liked. But once the paper was sent off, nothing more was asked of him.[59]

Even if there had been difficulties, the School of Hygiene is no great distance from St Mary's where bacteriologists abounded. Why was Fleming himself not called upon to help?

And so the matter rested until 1934 when Lewis Holt joined the staff of the Inoculation Department. He was a chemist by training. After some work for Wright on the causation of scurvy and with Fleming on staphylococcal toxoid, he was asked by the latter if he would like to add his name to the rapidly lengthening list of those who had attempted to purify and concentrate penicillin.

In any ordinary laboratory Fleming would have sat down with Holt and told him what Ridley and Craddock had been doing 6 years previously in his own laboratory. Fleming did no such thing. According to Holt, Clutterbuck's paper was mentioned and he was told to read it. But nothing whatever was said about the work of Ridley and Craddock. In fact, he never heard about it until long afterwards.

Holt made no attempt to concentrate mould juice by vacuum distillation but made use of the fact that penicillin was known by this time to be soluble in organic solvents. He used amyl acetate for this purpose. This possesses the great advantage that it does not mix with water. It was accordingly added to the mould juice after its pH had been adjusted to 5–6 with acid. The mixture was then shaken and the amyl acetate freed from the broth in a separating funnel. The amyl acetate was then shaken with a weak solution of sodium bicarbonate in water at a pH of about 8·0. Some of the penicillin went into solution in the bicarbonate. But there were heavy losses in the process due, almost certainly, to the bicarbonate being too alkaline.

Like all the rest, Holt soon lost his enthusiasm for penicillin, stopped work and never published his results. He tells me that it was the extreme instability of the substance that prompted him to do this. Fleming seems to have made no attempt to persuade him to carry on with the work. As it turned out this was unfortunate because Holt's method was very similar to that which was eventually used.

Except for some abortive attempts by Dr R. Reid in America,[69] nothing further seems to have been done until 1939, when Prof. Howard Florey and Dr E. Chain at Oxford, evolved a method that finally solved the problem. I will refer to this later.

Chapter 6

The Villain of the Piece

The fact that penicillin appeared to be devoid of toxicity and that it could prevent the growth of several species of disease-producing microbes naturally suggested that it might be valuable as a chemotherapeutic agent. But in view of the fact that the stable, concentrated solution essential for the treatment of deep-seated infections was not forthcoming, Fleming was naturally limited as to what he could do. This amounted to no more than the application of crude mould juice to surface or accessible infections.

The first patient was Craddock. His antrum had become infected by a diphtheroid organism that was sensitive to penicillin. He irrigated the antrum himself twice a day with mould juice. It had no effect on the infection.[16] A little later, mould juice was used for the treatment of an infected amputation stump in the wards of the hospital but apparently without any useful effect. He had better luck with the next case. Rogers, one of his assistants, had contracted a pneumococcal infection of his eye. It was required so that he could take part in a shooting match. This being a form of sport much favoured by Fleming, he treated the eye with mould juice. The infection disappeared and Rogers was able to take his place in the team. Who won, has not, unfortunately, been recorded.[71]

If anything else was done along these lines, it cannot have amounted to much because the only references are in papers published in the following years, Thus, in the original paper describing the discovery, Fleming mentioned 'experiments in connection with its value are in progress'[24] and again, in 1931, 'It is likely that it (penicillin) or a chemical of a similar nature will be used in the treatment of septic wounds'.[25] A year later he said in another paper, 'It has been used in a number of septic wounds and has certainly appeared to be superior to dressings containing potent chemicals'.[27] Some time later, in 1941, he said, 'About 1930, it was used as a dressing on a few septic wounds with favourable results, but as in peace time septic wounds are uncommon in hospital, and as the potency of penicillin rapidly disappears on keeping, the therapeutic aspect of this substance was dropped.[32] and finally, in the Harben Lectures of 1945, there is a passage whose construction is so unfortunate that it must have been an uncorrected short-hand note, which reads as follows, 'We tried it tentatively on a few old sinuses in the hospital and although the reports were favourable there was nothing miraculous. When we asked the surgeons if they had any septic cases they never had any, and then perhaps when they asked us if we had any and our whole supply had become inert.'[34]

As will be gathered from these quotations, Fleming evidently did think that penicillin might be of value when used locally, even though his attempts to employ it can only be described as feeble.

It seems unfortunate that Fleming should have behaved in this way because even crude mould juice was shown, in the early 1930s, to have considerable value. My friend Dr C. G. Paine treated two types of infection in the Royal Infirmary in Sheffield.

The first were chronic staphylococcal infections of the skin. Three patients were given local applications every 4 hours for a week, and although the infecting organisms were all shown to be sensitive to penicillin there was no improvement.

The second were infections of the eye. Two cases of gono-coccal ophthalmitis in children were cured in 2 to 3 days. So too was a case of staphylococcal conjunctivitis. The organism was sensitive to penicillin, but that infecting a second case was found to be resistant and there was no improvment in the clinical condition. This must have been the first time that a naturally resistant strain was detected.

The eighth case was the most instructive. The patient had had a penetrating injury of the eye and there was a severe pneumococcal infection of the conjunctival sac that prevented operation for the removal of a foreign body. The pneumococcus was sensitive to penicillin, and irrigation of the conjunctiva with mould juice brought about clearance of the infection within 48 hours, so that the operation could be performed and the eye was saved.

Paine did not publish this work but it is referred to by Florey, who was his chief at the time, in the monograph the latter published after the war.[40] Although Paine had been a student at St Mary's, I doubt whether Fleming knew of this work. He certainly never referred to it, nor did Paine continue with it. The latter left the Royal Infirmary shortly afterwards to work in the isolation hospital attached to the Jessop Hospital for Women. Here he encountered patients with puerperal fever, but like us in London made no attempt to use penicillin for the treatment of this disease.

If Fleming himself did very little towards establishing the value of penicillin when applied locally, he did at least record the fact that he had tried it and that he evidently had some belief in it. It is also probable that for a few months following the discovery he may have thought of it as a valuable agent for the treatment of deep-seated infections in which it would have to be carried to the infected area by the blood stream. Indeed, this was one of the reasons for the attempts of Ridley and Craddock to concentrate the penicillin in mould juice. But it is extremely difficult to believe that this mood of optimism persisted for very long.

There is certainly no reference to this method of treatment in any of the papers or speeches he made in the following years. In fact, he said very little about penicillin as a chemotherapeutic agent; so much so that when, in 1932, he had to give his Presidential Address to the Section of Pathology of the Royal Society of Medicine, an occasion when, allowed a full hour, the speaker discourses on a subject that particularly interests him and on which he is an authority, Fleming chose lysozyme. Even when the subject more directly concerned chemotherapy, Fleming generally ignored the opportunity. The first to provide one was a paper read in 1931 at a combined meeting of the Sections of Surgery and Pathology at the Royal Society of Medicine, and the title indicates its scope: 'On the indications for and the value of the intravenous use of germicides'. But although he dealt with such substances as eusol, monsol, quinine, mercuric chloride, mercurochrome, sanocrysin, flavine, gentian violet, neosalvarsan and hypertonic saline, he never mentioned penicillin.[26] This is the best example of an opportunity missed. But there were others in papers published in the *British Dental Journal* in 1931,[25] the *Journal of Pathology and Bacteriology* in 1932,[27] and in the *Proceedings of the Royal Society of Medicine* in 1939,[29] 1940[30, 31] and 1941.[32] In none is there even a hint of the possible use of penicillin for infections such as pneumonia, meningitis or osteomyelitis.

I am not alone in thinking this. Florey drew attention to it in 1944,[38] as did Colebrook in 1956 when he wrote, 'At that time (1929), Fleming seems to have had in his mind only the local application of penicillin'.[11] More recently a much younger bacteriologist, Dr W. D. Foster, has written, 'On the evidence, it is hard to believe that Fleming had any conception of the therapeutic possibilities of penicillin'.[43] What is more, those who were most closely associated with him during the early developmental phases of penicillin are of the same opinion. Ridley has repeatedly said much the same thing and Craddock, who knew him better than any of us, said in a letter written soon after Fleming's death, 'He thought it had possibilities in 1928 or early 1929, and he mentioned this in his original paper. But the instability, the cost of production and the very impure product convinced Flem that there was very little future in the stuff. His opinion of penicillin became very hardened after our failures to refine and preserve it. And so he classified it with lysozyme and regarded it as hopeless.' This opinion seems to have persisted until 1933 when Rogers became his assistant. He has told me, 'Flem did not imagine that penicillin would be used in the way it is now.' And finally Maclean, who not only shared his laboratory but collaborated in research on penicillin, said much the same thing to me in 1958, shortly before he left this country to die in his native New Zealand.

If, following his original optimism, Fleming began to have doubts about penicillin, there were four very good reasons for them.

The first was, in a sense, psychological. Too many substances were already known that seemed to be quite as valuable as penicillin but which had already been shown to be useless in practice. There were, for example, a number of other antibiotics, penicillin being by no means the first to be discovered. As early as 1887, Pasteur and Joubert had observed that the growth of anthrax bacilli could be prevented by what they called 'common bacteria'. And Prof. Gratia, a firm friend of Fleming, had shown in 1924, that certain species of actinomycetes could produce antibiotics acting on other organisms. But the best known was pyocyanase produced by *Pseudomonas pyocyanea* which could prevent growth of anthrax and diphtheria bacilli. It had been used clinically for many years, but it had been found to be practically useless.

There were also the arsenical compounds that Colebrook and I had been using. Their credentials were quite as good as those of penicillin. Fleming knew this and he also knew that they were proving to be useless. If this were not enough, there were the bacteriophages, viruses that multiply inside bacteria and destroy them but are harmless to patients. One of Fleming's best friends, Dr Arthur Compton, was giving them to patients with dysentery in Alexandria but with very little useful effect. There was precious little in all this to encourage anyone to spend much time on penicillin.

The second reason, pure conjecture on my part but I have little doubt that it must have influenced Fleming, was the fact that Craddock had found that staphylococci could become resistant to penicillin after only short exposure to it. It would take too long to describe exactly how the experiment was carried out but the classical method was employed in which the organisms were 'trained' by growing them in broth containing penicillin in too small amounts to kill them. As a result of only three such passages, the Hall strain of staphylococci became able to multiply in broth containing mould juice at a dilution of only 1/100 (but not in 1/10) whereas before treatment in this way, it had been inhibited in all dilutions up to and including 1/400.[16]

For some unknown reason this experiment was never published or, so far as I know, ever referred to by Fleming, and it was not until 1941 that the Oxford team confirmed it by showing that the sensitivity of staphylococci could be decreased a thousand-fold by this method.[1]

TABLE 1. TO SHOW THE FALL IN TITRE OF MOULD JUICE WHEN KEPT AT ROOM TEMPERATURE

	Titre 1/640 pH 8·5				
	pH unaltered		pH adjusted to 6·0		pH adjusted to 6·0 and tubes filled with CO_2
	not waxed	waxed	not waxed	waxed	waxed
7 days					
Titre	1/80	1/80	1/320	1/320	1/320
pH	8·5	8·5	6·5	6·0	6·0
14 days					
Titre	1/80	1/80	1/160	1/320	1/320
pH	8·5	8·5	7·0	6·5	6·5
28 days					
Titre	<1/10	<1/10	1/160	1/160	1/160

This form of resistance is due to mutation and it is now known that staphylococci seldom acquire it while causing infections in patients under treatment. Fleming could not have known this. What he did know was the standard doctrine of the time; that resistance can be acquired under treatment, that once resistance has been acquired it is a permanent characteristic and that if such an organism produces infection, treatment by the chemo-therapeutic agent is valueless.

The third reason was that although Ridley and Craddock had worked out a method for the small-scale partial purification of penicillin, it was obvious that it was much too clumsy for its production in any quantity. A good chemist might have suggested better methods based on what had been learned, but I doubt whether Fleming realized this. Furthermore, Fleming was temperamentally unsuited to large-scale work of any kind. He was used to working by himself with micro-methods. It was also far beyond the capacity of the laboratory where space was at a premium.

The fourth and in my opinion by far the most important reason was that penicillin was so extremely unstable. Fleming quoted an experiment in his first paper, which showed that when kept at room temperature the antibacterial activity of mould juice had practically disappeared in 15 days. Although he mentioned that if the pH was dropped from the original 9·0 to 6·8 the activity persisted longer, he did not say for how long.

Several attempts seem to have been made to get over this difficulty. They tried to detect an enzyme that might inactivate it, but failed. They thought it might be the action of light and kept mould juice in black tubes, but this did not improve matters. The third idea arose from the fact that all the glassware in those days was markedly alkaline and that this caused the pH to rise so much that even when acidified, inactivation could still occur. They therefore used tubes lined with wax. They even went further and filled some of them with carbon dioxide. This experiment is sufficiently interesting to merit a table giving the results. It not only shows the effect of pH on the longevity of penicillin, but that as early as 1929, they knew a good deal more about it[16] than the laconic statement in the paper would indicate.

Nevertheless, although Clutterbuck and his colleagues were able to keep penicillin for longer periods, the fact remained that unless it could be kept indefinitely, ready for use when needed, it was very nearly useless as a chemotherapeutic agent.

I should perhaps add that expedients that would be employed almost automatically nowadays had either not been thought of or were not available. Deep freeze cabinets could not be bought until the 1950s. When dry ice became available I do not know, but in 1929 the largest amount that could be obtained at St Mary's was a stick about the size of a pencil produced by the hospital pharmacist for the treatment of warts. Freeze drying under vacuum or lyophilization as it is sometimes called, was quite unknown. The first time I became aware of it was when its value for the preservation of cultures was demonstrated by a number of speakers at the International Congress of Microbiology in London in 1936. In any event, the only vacuum pump owned by the department was a hand-operated model of ancient vintage which was quite unsuitable for such a purpose. But it was, in the end, this method that saved the day for penicillin, all the early preparations being preserved in this way.

These four reasons were well known to Fleming by the summer of 1929 and it is very difficult to believe that, with them in mind, he could have had much faith in penicillin as a chemotherapeutic agent. Small wonder that he did virtually nothing to ascertain the value of penicillin during the next 11 years.

This inactivity, or to put it more charitably, lack of anything tangible after 11 years, was a serious matter when Fleming became a celebrity and was asked the obvious questions; whether he had anticipated from the beginning that penicillin would eventually prove to be so valuable and, if he had, why he had not pursued the matter to the bitter end instead of stopping when he did.

Fleming, being no fool, knew perfectly well that to have answered these questions in detail would have quickly landed him in a morass of technicalities, almost certain to be misunderstood by his questioners, from which he would have had great difficulty in extricating himself. Very wisely he parried them by saying something to the effect that he himself was not a chemist, that no chemist had produced a preparation suitable for injection, and that without such material he had been unable to ascertain what value, if any, the substance possessed.

When, however, his biography came to be written 13 years after this, there was so little drama about this *apologia* that the novelist who wrote it evidently felt it incumbent on him to introduce a little. Being already provided with a hero, he added a villain to the cast. The unfortunate individual chosen to act the part was Wright.

His being cast for the part seems to have depended on the

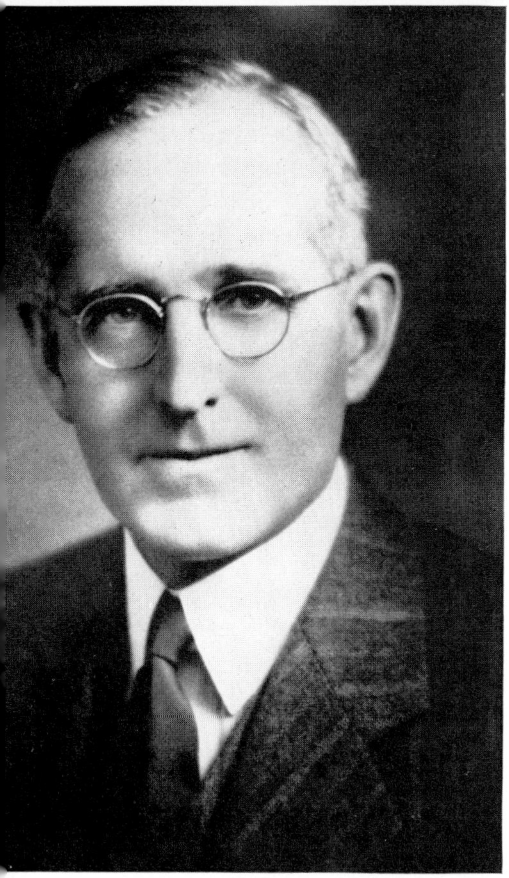

VII. J. G. Fitzgerald.

Mould growing in the bottles used for the production of penicillin in 1944.

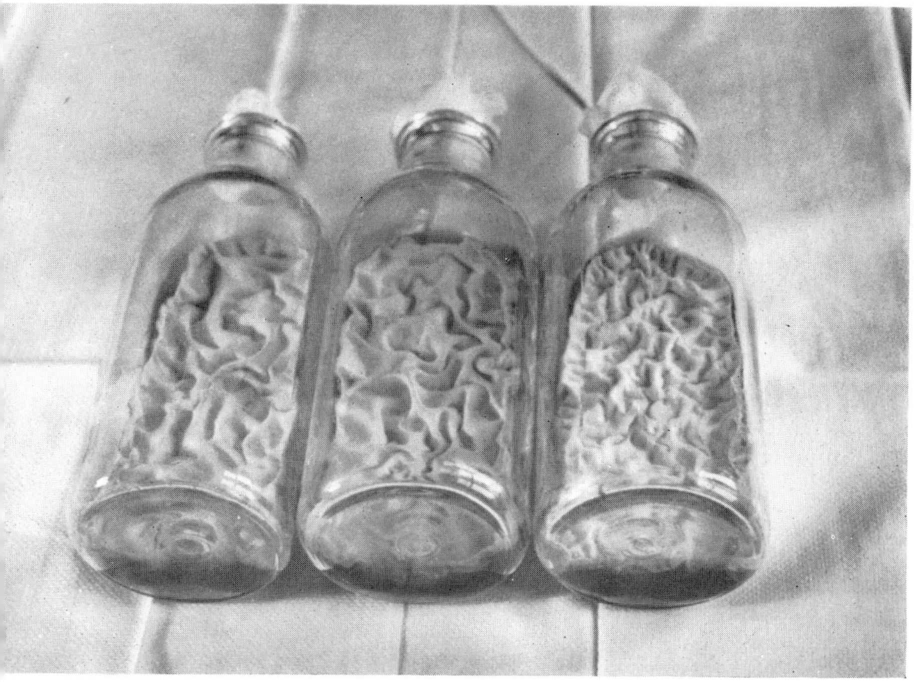

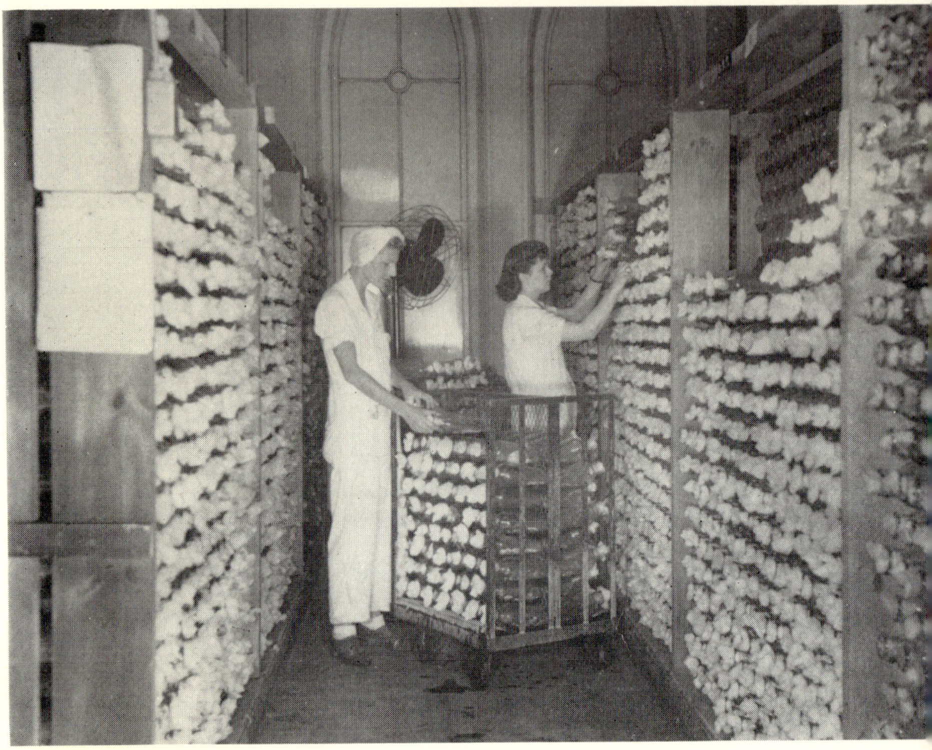

VIII. Incubation room for the production of penicillin.

Processing the bottles after harvesting the medium containing penicillin.

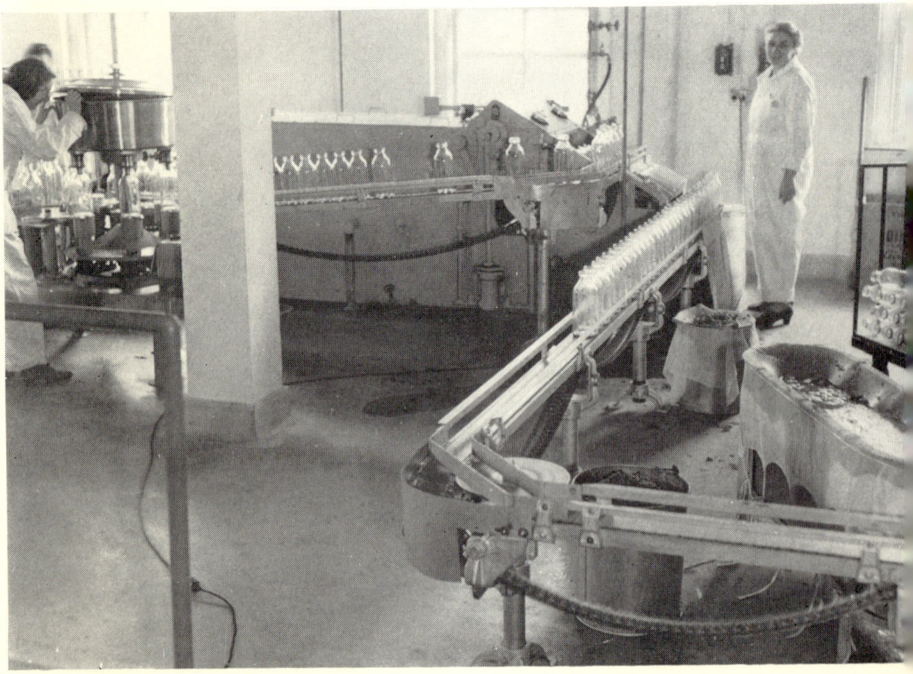

supposition that he was an implacable enemy of chemotherapy and Maurois becomes almost lyrical in developing this theme. Thus, 'Wright could say again as he had said in 1912 that "the chemotherapy of human bacterial infections will never be possible" ' 'chemotherapy still inspired him with an invincible repugnance'; and, more directly relating to Fleming, 'all Wright's instincts were up in arms against penicillin'. But not only Wright, for the whole department would seem to have shared in the villainy if it were true that 'more especially was the atmosphere hostile in Wright's department'.

As a result of all this, any uninformed reader would be justified in assuming that for the best part of 11 years the whole of the Inoculation Department had barely been on speaking terms with Fleming, led by its Chief as an *éminence grise* who so loathed chemotherapy in general and penicillin in particular that he had been prepared to hinder Fleming as much as he could. It is accordingly not very surprising that in a book published as recently as 1965 it is stated, 'his Chief, Sir Almroth Wright not only failed to encourage, but actively attempted to obstruct him'.[3]

It is, however, astonishing how little evidence Maurois produces in support of his contention. All that I can find in the Biography are three statements. The first is a quotation from what is presumably a letter from Sir Henry Dale in which it is stated that if Fleming had been working in a laboratory under someone 'willing to accept and even to find attractive', the fact that the chemotherapy of bacterial infections would eventually be possible, more rapid progress might have been made. The second is that Wright objected to Fleming's suggestion in the original paper that penicillin might be of value for the local treatment of surface infections. The third is so unsatisfactory that I am doubtful whether it should be included at all. It is a reference to a conversation Fleming had had with a Dr J. Taylor who is not further identified, in the course of which the latter had said that Fleming had been fortunate in having Wright's backing. Maurois fails to mention for what purpose the backing was required but implies that it was the development of penicillin and gives Fleming's reply, 'No, on the contrary'.

Maurois also fails to describe what form Wright's opposition took or at what stage it occurred but suggests that, whatever it was, the end result was that Fleming could not hope for more money or assistance.

Much of the drama that Maurois succeeds in imparting was, I suppose, founded on what Dale had said and which was repeated in somewhat similar vein in a contribution to the obituary in the *British Medical Journal*. In it he said, 'neither the time when the discovery was made, nor, perhaps, the scientific atmosphere of the laboratory in which he worked, was propitious to such further enterprise as its development would have needed. Repeated failure had caused opinion then to harden, almost into a settled conviction, against the possibility of a successful chemotherapy of the common bacterial infections. Sir Almroth Wright himself had no belief in such a possibility.'[18]

Having been President of the Royal Society, Dale's opinions naturally carried great weight with Maurois. But this does not necessarily guarantee their accuracy. He was an octogenarian at the time whose principal activities had concerned pharmacology. He was certainly no bacteriologist. Nor was he a great friend of Wright's; in fact I have reason to believe that he had a low opinion of Wright's abilities. He never visited the Inoculation Department and could have known little about its internal affairs. I doubt whether he would have said what he did had he known that for 5 years two members of the laboratory were studying chemotherapy and, at one time, no less than five.

In his search for a scapegoat, Maurois grossly exaggerated the importance of Dale's comparatively innocuous remarks. In so doing, he revealed his ignorance of the ways of research laboratories the world over. It is probable, in fact almost certain, that Fleming did ask Wright for assistance of some kind. But persuading one's chief to give one more space, more materials and above all, more staff, is generally more difficult than making discoveries. If, then, he did not get what he asked for, Fleming met the same fate that comes at least once in the career of every research worker who is really earning his salary. If he is wise, he recognizes it as part of the game, lets the dust die down and tries again. He may have better luck next time. But no matter how infuriated he may be, he – or his biographer if he merits one – does not denounce his chief as a scoundrel who is doing his best to hinder him.

In any event, refusal of assistance is a very long way from deliberate obstruction. Had there been anything of this nature it is a little difficult to see how I could have avoided noticing it. During some at least of the material time I worked only about 10 feet away from Wright, in almost the exact position that Sir Gerald Kelly must have occupied when painting the portrait that is now in the library of the Wright Fleming Institute. Here I was in the midst of everything, and as Wright had nowhere else to discuss even matters of high policy I heard or soon learned about nearly everything that was going on. But there was never even the slightest hint that Wright was trying to prevent Fleming's work on penicillin.

What is more, I was working with Colebrook on the very subject that Wright, according to Maurois, found so repugnant. But neither of us, nor Ridley or Craddock, were ever made to feel that we were doing something he would rather we did not do. In fact, he actually went out of his way to help us by bringing back with him, following a visit to Paris, a rabbit from the Pasteur Institute which had been infected with the spirochaetes of syphilis so that we could find an answer to an important chemotherapeutic question, the time taken by the arsenicals to kill them. We never did, nor did we infect ourselves. But it is a little difficult to believe that an elderly gentleman would have gone to the trouble of including amongst his baggage a large wicker basket containing a rabbit with syphilis of its scrotum, and be prepared to satisfy the inevitable curiosity of the customs officials at Dover, if he loathed chemotherapy so much that he was prepared to obstruct a favourite pupil in his attempts to exploit a discovery.

Nevertheless, there was hostility in the Inoculation Department – but only to that form of chemotherapy that involved the use of general protoplasmic poisons such as the antiseptics. Here Fleming was an even more vehement opponent than any of us. But there was no hostility to chemotherapy with more creditable compounds such as the arsenicals and, when they appeared, the sulphonamides. The nearest Wright ever got to hostility was to have doubt about them. And we have it on the authority of Colebrook that after publishing his paper in *The Lancet* in1927 he took very little interest in the subject. In fact, as I have already pointed out, he took very little interest in anything except immunity in vitro and logic from then onwards.

Thus Maurois completely misinterpreted the situation in the Inoculation Department; so much so that there is no evidence whatever to suggest that Wright was responsible for the 11 years of inactivity on the part of his hero. But there was, for all that, a villain. It was penicillin itself that should have been cast for the part. Its similarity to other agents known to be useless, its ability to induce resistance on the part of previously sensitive organisms, its paucity in the fluids in which it was produced, and above all its instability, made it the real villain of the piece. And what is more, it played its part better than did Wright.

Chapter 7

Mothers and Molecules

The period lasting from September 1928, when penicillin was discovered, until the end of 1931, by which time whatever hopes Fleming may have had of the work at the School of Hygiene were beginning to fade, may be regarded as the first phase in the history of penicillin. For the next 9 years, until the first of the Oxford papers was published in the summer of 1940, penicillin remained no more than another of the antibiotics, the first of which had been discovered as long before as 1887. In all probability it was classed in the minds of those who thought about it at all as no better and no worse than pyocyanase, which had proved to be clinically useless long before.

Nevertheless, dormant though penicillin might be, chemotherapy as a science was very much alive; so much so that the first of the sulphonamides, whose introduction into medicine can be regarded as the birth of chemotherapy as we know it today, was actually patented about the beginning of this period on November 7, 1931. It was several years before the discoveries that followed were applied to the treatment of disease to any great extent. But when they were, they had immense consequences. It is this phase in the history of chemotherapy with which this and the following chapter is concerned.

Having been fortunate enough to see the discovery of penicillin and the early stages of its development, I was equally fortunate to witness and even play some part in the events during this second phase in the development of the science. This, too, came about by sheer chance and without premeditation on my part, being due to nothing more than the attempts Colebrook and I were making to cure puerperal fever.

This disease is almost unknown nowadays but in 1931 was still a matter of serious concern to obstetricians everywhere. They had begun to realize during the mid-20s that it was still as common as it had been half a century before, but the incidence and death rates from such diseases as typhoid and dysentery had fallen dramatically over the same period. Why had that of puerperal fever remained so persistently horizontal? Surely something could be done to bring the curve down towards the baseline?

The obstetricians themselves could do very little. They were too busy making a living. Nor did they know where to start. Ministries of Health, too, were at a loss but felt that it was time they did something. They reacted as do all government departments when faced with an apparently insoluble problem. With singular unanimity, wherever they were, they appointed a committee to investigate it. It usually consisted of the more vocal but not necessarily best-informed obstetricians in the community, public health officers whose main qualification was that they knew no bacteriology, and a statistician who had probably never seen a patient with the disease.

The results of their deliberations could have been predicted. They reported what everyone already knew, that puerperal fever occurred in their community, that quite a number of women died of it, that it was a problem and that further investigations were in progress. None of them had the courage to admit that such investigations amounted to no more than the gathering of yet more statistics and that no one had the slightest idea where the microbes came from, how they got into the birth canal and why some patients died and others recovered. Still less did they know how to prevent it.

It was only too obvious that something more than a government committee was required if puerperal fever was to be dealt with. Strange as it may seem, it was, and within 10 years. But largely by the efforts of men and women who were not on these committees.

The process began in the summer of 1928 while Colebrook

was away in Breslau working in the laboratory of Prof. Carl Prausnitz, who ended his days as Dr Giles and a much-loved general practitioner in Ventnor. Colebrook had gone to stay with him in order to perfect his German. This was advisable because so much of the fundamental work had been done in that country, and its literature still required perusal if one was to keep up with progress. And as if to emphasize the importance he attached to it, he gave me the two enormous volumes of Muret Sander's dictionary as a wedding present a year or two later.

Before departing he had planned almost every moment of my time for me. I was to do such and such an experiment on such and such a day, and so forth. But he omitted to plan my spare time. I therefore felt free to attend when I was summoned to a meeting held one evening in the house of Sir D'Arcy Power in Chandos Place. Here I encountered most of the obstetric talent of London around one of the largest dinner tables I have ever seen.

It transpired that Queen Charlotte's Maternity Hospital had decided to move. For the best part of a century it had inhabited the building in the Marylebone Road that is now an annexe of St Dunstan's. There was no operating theatre, and emergency operations such as Caesarian sections had to be done in the labour ward hastily converted for the purpose. But there was nowhere to build something more suitable. Nor was it at all certain that a mother-to-be deposited in the lift would reach the labour ward on the top of the building before the great event, for it was an ancient hydraulic contraption given to bouts of asthma and frequently out of action altogether. Practically everything else about the place was equally out of date.

I had known the place for some time and could sympathize with them. I had done my obstetrics there while still a student. This necessitated staying a fortnight in a hostel in Cosway Street 100 yards away, being continuously on call so that when the bell in the passage rang loudly to signify that another member of the human race was about to appear, we could drop whatever we were doing and even get out of bed and dress in order to race across the Marylebone Road in time for the ceremony. Since large numbers of midwives were also being trained, the six medical students were seldom called upon to take an active part in the process. Even when they were it amounted to very little, because obstetrics in those days was largely a matter of exhortations to the mother and most of them came from the formidable female in charge of the labour ward.

In view of the fact that I was to be a member of its staff for 5 years, I ought to have taken more interest in the proceedings. I did not know this at the time. But L. J. Davis was one of my fellow students. He eventually became Professor of Medicine in the University of Glasgow and was, like me, more interested in the scientific aspects of medicine than in obstetrics. The two of us therefore tended to leave midwifery to the midwives while we talked pathology in a corner.

In any event they were not inspiring performances. The place was overcrowded, little regard was paid to sterility and anaesthesia was conspicuous by its absence.

Later, when I became Colebrook's assistant, I used to visit it to help them with their bacteriological investigations. We also gave transfusions if the patient was infected. The wearing of white gowns being still uncommon, we usually did the operation in our shirt sleeves. On one such occasion a student from St Mary's, who I happened to know, seemed beside himself with ill-concealed merriment. Not until the operation was over did I discover the reason; a cleaner's label which was still attached by safety pins to my waistcoat looked suspiciously like a pawn ticket.

Since the hospital was past redemption, they had decided to get out and build a new one. In those days the process was much simpler than it is now. Instead of petitioning, begging, pleading or lobbying the Ministry of Health to provide the money, one simply bought a site and built the hospital, and moreover the sort of hospital one wanted, not what the Ministry's architects thought would be good for you. The money required for this exercise was collected in the best way one could devise, but it was generally forthcoming.

As a first step in this process the governing body had bought a site in the Goldhawk Road in faraway Chiswick on which a brand new hospital was to be built. But it had also decided that it would do something active towards the conquest of puerperal fever by building a small hospital for the treatment of cases of the disease, and a laboratory next door where they could be properly investigated.

This was to be proceeded with as soon as possible and would, it was hoped, demonstrate to the world how progressive was Queen Charlotte's. In this way Mr Seymour Leslie, their professional collector, would be provided with the armament for the persuasion of possible donors of money to produce sufficient for the building of their main hospital.

Up to this point, my presence at the meeting seemed superfluous. But before very long I found myself advising men who had been my examiners only 4 years previously how to build their new hospital and, what is perhaps more remarkable, found them listening to me.

Then came the question: Who should run the research laboratory? There was only one answer – my chief, Colebrook. But as he was away in Germany, nothing could be done at that time.

When he returned he was, as I had expected, pained that the meeting had been held without him, and even more pained that he had been represented by me. In fact so pained, that for a time I doubted whether he would accept the appointment. But take it he did and I was to go with him. The third member of the staff was to be my friend Dr R. M. Fry, who had been Wright's assistant for some time and needed a change if he was to retain his sanity.

In due course the Isolation Block, as the new hospital was called, was ready for occupation. It was a luxurious building with wide balconies looking out on the gardens that were legacies from the large houses on the site. A little later the laboratories were finished, and we moved in on January 1, 1931.

Since Colebrook never did anything by halves and this was his first independent command, every detail of the building had been planned with the utmost care. The doorhandles, for example, were constructed in such a way that one could open the door without using the hands; the elbows, chin or even the eyebrows would suffice. The opening of the windows was a more serious problem. They were ordinary metal casements, but so orthodox a method as leaning over the bench and pulling the handle down was considered to be unsuitable. Something on the bench might have got knocked over. After prolonged consultations between Colebrook, the architects, the engineers and, of course, the makers of the windows, a contraption was at last evolved. Its main feature was a long pole with which one unscrewed the window while standing on the far side of the bench. But as the pole usually got lost, it was difficult to work; we seldom opened the windows, and never knocked things over, it was never used – not even by its inventor.

It was the library, however, that had received the most loving care. Its floor was a particularly resilient specimen of cork carpet, and much more luxurious than the battleship linoleum which had to suffice for the rest of the building. The exact tone of the stain used for the pine bookshelves had required prolonged research. But it was the walls that had received the most attention. The off-white suitable for the rest of the building was considered to be much too dull, and after endless experiments a delicate greenish blue was finally chosen.

Although the walls looked lovely they were very bare, and accordingly pictures were suggested. At first it seemed that the proper course was to hang portraits of the great bacteriological pioneers, and a singularly dull steel engraving of Pasteur was duly installed. A second was a pencil drawing of Wright by an eminent Royal Academician. This was even less successful because the sitting seemed to have occurred at a time when the subject was in a very bad temper, so that the portrait was only just recognizable. Further additions to the portrait gallery came to an end at this point. The only available portrait of Koch made him look like a prosperous business man, which he was not. We also felt that, as we were studying puerperal fever, Semmelweis ought to be included. But even the best picture made him look so like a hunting squire back from a long run (and too tired to remove his riding boots and overcoat) that his inclusion would have required too much explanation. The only other candidate was Ehrlich, but as he had been responsible for the arsenicals that had not been particularly helpful, we could hardly number him amongst our patron saints. But there still remained a lot of greenish blue.

The suggestion was then made that, as a purely temporary measure until one or other of us won a Nobel Prize and with the money could afford to have a portrait painted, we would have pictures instead. As I was the only member with connections with High Art, I was told to do something about it. Holding out the bait that, as we frequently had to show round rich visitors with a view to their becoming donors to the hospital, they might take a fancy to some of the pictures on the walls so that sales might result, I was able to obtain quite a number of etchings and woodcuts from friends of my sister who, like her, were students at a College of Art.

Suspecting that Colebrook had envisaged not more than two or three choice specimens that he had seen and approved, I was greatly disturbed to find that my sister evidently had too many friends because no less than six of them submitted samples of their work. The omission of only one of the young artists from the display might have been disastrous if they ever came to see us. All that I could do in the circumstances was to select one of each artist's works, hang them one Monday morning, and hope for the best.

Colebrook never quite recovered from the shock he sustained when he came in for lunch, but as they had cost us nothing he could not express the feelings that were uppermost in his mind. He was always ill at ease whenever visitors congratulated us on our picture gallery. But whoever they were, none of them ever showed signs of wanting to buy any works of the artists represented, and the walls are still waiting for the Nobel Laureate.

Although we had, if anything, too many pictures, we were very short of money. Colebrook and I were paid by the Medical Research Council who also gave a grant towards our expenses. But Fry's salary had to be found by the hospital and we needed more staff. To make matters worse there was a depression, and things seemed likely to get worse rather than better. The Rockefeller Foundation was, accordingly, approached for help and Dr Gregg, its European representative who lived in Paris, signified his intention of calling upon us.

I was not present at the ceremony, but I was never doubtful about its outcome. If there was one person likely to impress a possible benefactor, it was Colebrook. His missionary zeal, his patent honesty and his mastery of the subject, conveyed what was undoubtedly true, the impression of a dedicated worker out to benefit humanity. No one else that I knew could have created the same image.

Even so, the battle was by no means over when Dr Gregg departed. Long afterwards it emerged that his colleagues had been more than doubtful. But Gregg won the day and we were promised the tidy sum of £5,000 a year for 7 years. He used to come and see us about once a year and it was in this way that I got to know a very charming individual. With the money provided in this way and by the Bernhard Baron Trustees who contributed the cost of the building, it was possible to appoint Colebrook's sister Dora, and Elizabeth White, both bacteriologists, and Albert Fuller, a biochemist.

It was in this way that Queen Charlotte's Hospital became, almost without realizing it, the world headquarters for research on puerperal fever and, for a time at least, of chemotherapy.

Up to this point I have said very little about the disease we were studying or the applications of our work to medicine as a whole. First let us consider puerperal fever itself. Its causation is comparatively simple. After the baby is born the uterus, which consists almost entirely of muscle, contracts to a much smaller size. The membrane that lines it remains intact and protects the tissues lying beneath. But this membrane does not cover the site where the placenta was attached. This is now a large, raw area and is, for all practical purposes, an open wound. As it is some distance from the outside world it is protected from the many microbes that may be present in the environment. But like all open wounds, blood oozes from the vessels in the raw area, and clots as soon as it reaches the uterine cavity. The serum that is produced in this way not only fills the cavity but drains out through the neck or cervix of the uterus to reach the vagina, and eventually the outside of the body. Here it encounters the many species of microbes that may be present on the skin, clothing or bedding. The great majority are killed by substances in the serum and, even if they are not, they are unlikely to grow in it. But, unfortunately, some microbes can grow in serum and with great rapidity. The streptococci are particularly liable to do this. The result is that, even if there are only a few streptococci in the vagina or on the skin outside, they can grow along the film of serum to reach the interior of the uterus and the raw area of the placental site. From then on, puerperal fever is inevitable.

There is no reason to doubt that something of this nature still occurs. But thanks to the antibiotics it is generally allowed to go no further. The patient is given penicillin as soon as the symptoms appear, and recovers within a day or so. But before the advent of modern chemotherapeutic agents it was a very different matter. Infection occurred of a severity the modern doctor never encounters or even hears about because so few of his teachers have ever seen a fully developed case.

At the time we went to Queen Charlotte's it was sufficiently common to kill one, two or even more per thousand women who had babies. Many more had the disease in milder form but the illness might be very prolonged before they recovered. All in all, puerperal fever was a severe illness with a high mortality, and dreaded by both mothers and obstetricians alike.

The symptoms usually started with a high temperature on the third day after delivery and before very long the patient was seriously ill. About half were caused by streptococci, which are somewhat unusual in being unable to multiply in the presence of oxygen. The resulting illness was comparatively mild but some of the patients had chills every day, sometimes for a month or more. But only 5 per cent of them died.

The real problem were the patients infected by another variety of streptococci, usually referred to as haemolytic streptococci but whose official name is *Streptococcus pyogenes*. Those infected by this microbe were in serious danger from the beginning largely because it can grow so rapidly in the serum present in the birth canal after delivery. In about three-quarters of the patients, the infection was halted by the body defences soon after it reached the placental site. The patient might be quite ill, but she was not likely to die.

In the remainder, the microbe, aided by its production of an enzyme called fibrinolysin, took full advantage of its ability to spread through the tissues. When this occurred, the outlook for the patient was bleak. Spread of the microbe through the uterine wall meant that peritonitis was inevitable and there are few worse diseases than this. Almost as bad was the septicaemia that resulted if the microbe reached the blood vessels in the placental site for it could gain access to every other organ in the body. Very few patients with these complications recovered and even if they did, it had been a dreadful illness.

Although the prevention and cure of this disease were our main objectives, any lessons learnt as a result of our researches could be applied to the other much commoner infections caused by this microbe that have nothing to do with childbirth. These too can be controlled nowadays so easily by prompt treatment that few doctors realize the full potentialities for evil that the haemolytic streptococci exhibited 30 or 40 years ago. I therefore propose to say something more about them.

Tonsillitis and scarlet fever were the two commonest of the infections caused by these organisms. Although there was fever and difficulty in swallowing, most patients recovered without much trouble. But there was always the danger that the abilities of the organism to invade the tissues would complicate the matter. In consequence, abscesses of the throat commonly called quinsy, which had to be opened and could sometimes almost suffocate the patient, were not uncommon. The microbes might travel further to reach the glands in the neck and cause enormous swellings sometimes referred to as 'bull neck'. But the consequences were much more serious if the microbes travelled up the eustachian tube into the middle ear to cause otitis media; there must be many adults who are deaf today because of this. Far worse was it if they went further and got into the mastoid cells and, still worse, the meninges immediately adjacent, because meningitis caused by these organisms was an almost certain sentence of death.

If this had been all that a comparatively simple infection of the throat could lead to, it would have been quite enough, but as a result of a process still not completely understood, rheumatic fever and acute nephritis might follow such infections. Both were serious and often fatal diseases. And even when the patient recovered, a severely damaged kidney or heart might be the result. Many of the patients whose hearts were repaired by cardiac surgery after the war, were victims of a streptococcal infection in childhood.

Although a high proportion of the infections occurred in childhood, no age was immune. Many young adults died during the influenza pandemic of 1918–19 because streptococci invaded their lungs to cause a particularly vicious form of pneumonia. And many old people, usually in failing health already, died because they had contracted erysipelas, an infection of the skin, usually of the face. There was also constant danger that, whenever the skin was injured, streptococci would settle and produce infection of the wound. Even trivial injuries were quite sufficient to enable the organisms to reach the deeper tissues and grow. Many surgeons lost their lives because of pricks sustained at operations on infected patients. And one well-known artist died of streptococcal septicaemia because a model had scratched his face. If the wound was large, the danger became correspondingly greater. Burns and scalds were particularly liable to be infected by these organisms. So were the large gunshot wounds that were so common in France during the First World War. Indeed, it was largely as an outcome of this that Colebrook and I had become involved in a study of puerperal fever, which, in a sense, is a wound infection.

So seldom do severe infections by this microbe occur nowadays that it is difficult to convey to those who did not practise medicine in the 25 years between the wars, how much harm it did to the human race and how fortunate we are now to see so little of it. Nevertheless, although we at Queen Charlotte's were studying only one manifestation of its potentialities for evil, any lessons learned as a result of our work could be applied to the many other conditions for which it was also responsible. Thus, the Governors of an obstetric hospital may have been wiser than they perhaps realized when they determined to build a hospital and laboratory for the study of what may have seemed to be an exclusively obstetric disease.

Before I can proceed to describe our activities, it is necessary to say something about the microbe itself. Compared with most others it is comparatively simple, being no more than a sphere about 1/1,250 mm. in diameter. But unlike the staphylococci, which otherwise it resembles, it grows in the form of chains which may be made up of as many as twenty elements.

There are several varieties all producing semi-transparent colonies on agar culture plates containing blood. Some produce very little alteration in the blood and these are not likely to be harmful. But those of which I have been writing produce a very characteristic alteration in the blood near the colony. The red blood cells are so damaged by a substance called a haemolysin formed by the growing organisms, that they undergo dissolution or haemolysis as it is called. This gives the effect of a clear halo in the red opaque medium below and immediately surrounding the colony. It is for this reason that these organisms are generally called haemolytic streptococci.

Such, then, is the microbe with which we had to deal and the diseases for which it is responsible. Our first problem was the treatment of the patients. By this time the arsenicals, to which I have referred in Chapter 2, had revealed themselves to be frauds. They might be able to cure syphilis, but although they ought to have cured puerperal fever it was patent by this time that they could not. Even Colebrook was losing his enthusiasm for them. Unfortunately no other compound was available. Penicillin was, of course, discussed. It could not very well be ignored. But it was about this time that the paper by Clutterbuck, Lovell and Raistrick appeared. The mere fact that expert chemists in so well appointed a laboratory as the School of Hygiene had stopped studying it because it apparently disappeared into thin air when an ethereal solution was allowed to evaporate, sounded its death knell as far as we were concerned. We had neither the time nor the staff to pursue what seemed no more than a will o' the wisp, or as someone put it about that time, 'One of Flem's foolish fancies'.

The immunological methods that had been employed before

and after the war were barely mentioned. They provoked too much emotion. But this did not mean that immunology was finished, for someone, I suppose it must have been Wright, had had further ideas. Whoever it was had recalled that, in so far as the combating of microbes such as the streptococci was concerned, antibodies were not the only participants. They did not kill the microbes. They merely made them more palatable for the phagocytic cells to devour and digest them. If the appetites of these cells were not as ravenous as they ought to be, no wonder the patient could not kill the microbes and recover from the infection. What is more, it had only recently been shown that these cells could go off their food in streptococcal infections. Unfortunately, I was the person who had discovered it. I say 'unfortunately' because it was now proposed that, as phagocytic cells are present in abundance in the circulating blood of normal persons, we should treat the patients by giving them transfusions so that the more normal, more hungry phagocytic cells could take over the functions of the debilitated cells of the patient. I was hoist with my own petard, for although it was very doubtful whether deficiencies of these cells were responsible, or that those in a pint or so of normal human blood would make any difference, we were becoming so desperate that we could do nothing else but try.

Let no one think that they were ordinary transfusions. They were conducted with almost as much ceremony as a heart transplant operation today. Obtaining the blood was itself no light matter. Red Cross depots maintaining stocks of blood did not exist. One therefore conducted a search amongst friends and relatives of the patient for a suitable donor. If none could be found, the only recourse was a request to a public-spirited individual living in south London who had constituted himself a repository of information on donors all over London and, at any time of the day or night, would cheerfully find one and get him to the hospital within an hour or so. This meant that someone had to wait for his arrival for it was the height of bad form to keep him waiting.

The transfusion itself was highly abnormal. Citrate must not be added to the blood; it was said to injure the leucocytes. Nor could heparin be added; it was not yet available in a sufficiently pure condition. The only recourse was to defibrinate the blood. This meant that I sat on the floor beneath the couch and agitated the bottle into which the blood was drawn in such a way that the fibrin collected on a U-shaped glass rod inside the bottle. But this required no less than 20 minutes uninterrupted shaking at the end of which I was usually stiff with cramp.

The blood was then given to the patient. Not slowly as is done nowadays, but within 5 minutes or so by means of a syringe through a complicated system of tubes and stopcocks originally invented for the administration of arsenicals to patients with syphilis. Despite close observation, we never detected any signs of improvement.

This did not deter the sponsors. Normal blood evidently did not contain a sufficient number of leucocytes. Their numbers in the circulating blood can be doubled under certain circumstances, but the method chosen was the administration of sodium nucleinate. This approached the heroic because the package was invariably labelled, 'For veterinary use only' and the compound had to administered by intramuscular injection. The unfortunate donor then had to wait for 4 hours, during which time his bottom became increasingly painful, before his blood could be withdrawn. Heroic or not, this procedure never cured a patient.

Not to be defeated, the sponsors then told us that too many of the leucocytes had been lost by being collected in the clot. We must give whole, unclotted blood straight from the vein of a donor who had been dosed with sodium nucleinate. Blood clots so quickly that the ordinary apparatus could not be used. Fantastic expedients were employed to get over this difficulty. On one occasion we almost drowned ourselves with the ice cold water we used for chilling the blood to delay clotting. A German apparatus was produced but it proved a failure largely because even blood from a suitably prepared donor was unwilling to defy gravity by flowing uphill. In the end, the problem was solved by an apparatus of American origin. The first time we used it we suddenly realized that there was no way of telling which way the blood was flowing. This was awkward because some of the patients had large numbers of streptococci in their circulating blood. The instrument was promptly modified. But the psychological trauma to both of them must have been serious because the donor with his painful bottom had to lie within 12 inches of the patient, while the latter, already desperately ill, found herself in close proximity to a man she had never seen before. We gave a great many transfusions in this way but although we never lost a donor, I doubt whether we ever cured a patient.

I have described these futilities in some detail because I want to make it clear how serious were these illnesses and how ready we were to clutch at any straw that night help to keep the patient alive. Both Colebrook and I knew we were wasting our time. But this was the situation in which many doctors found themselves on countless occasions before modern chemotherapy was evolved. In the meanwhile, not knowing what else to do, all treatment was dropped for 2 or 3 years, and the best we could do for the patients was to give them magnificent nursing.

I suspect that the same passive attitude was adopted in other places. And when I was in Vienna about this time, I called to see Prof. Halban, one of the foremost European gynaecologists, and author with Dr Koeller of one of the best books on the morbid anatomy of puerperal fever. He told me that he treated his patients by giving them alcohol intravenously. When I protested that all this could do would be to make them drunk, he agreed with me, but smiled and added that it so improved their morale that they became better able to deal with the infection themselves. And so, 25 years after my father's death, the treatment of puerperal fever in both London and Vienna was fundamentally the same as he had given his patients. The only difference was that the brandy he would probably have prescribed for his patients was injected into the veins in Vienna. In London, it was still given by mouth.

If we could not cure puerperal fever, could we prevent it occurring at all? To do this required a great deal of information we did not possess at the time we went to Queen Charlotte's. Amongst other things, we did not know exactly which microbes caused some of the infections. We were not sure where any of them came from and even less did we know how they reached the patients. But without essential information on these matters, it was almost impossible to suggest methods for the prevention of the disease. To fill these gaps in our knowledge seemed a formidable undertaking at the time. But, strange as it may seem, they were filled before 5 years had passed; and with this to go on, the prevention of many cases of puerperal fever became practicable.

I do not propose to describe the whole business if only because it is a highly technical matter. But partly because those caused by the haemolytic streptococci were the most important and partly because the results obtained concerned a whole series of diseases that have nothing to do with childbirth, I propose to confine myself to these organisms.

Where these organisms came from was difficult to ascertain. We knew that they were comparatively common inhabitants of the throat and nose of normal persons, but it was also known that haemolytic streptococci might also be present in the vagina before delivery. Many obstetricians understandably thought it was these that had caused the infection when it made its appearance. There was a great deal of evidence to suggest that this had not occurred but, until it could be proved, no one knew how to prevent the disease. I was told to provide an answer.

I will not describe the blind trails we followed. But one day I was examining the colonies on a blood agar culture plate that had grown from a swab taken from the vagina of a pregnant woman who subsequently showed no signs of infection. There were a great many haemolytic streptococci on the plate. But unlike all previous specimens, the areas of haemolysis were not all the same size. Some were much larger than others. Nevertheless, the colonies themselves and the areas of haemolysis produced by both varieties superficially resembled strains that could cause puerperal fever.

Fortunately, what is now a classical paper by Dr Rebecca Lancefield of the Rockefeller Institute in New York had appeared shortly before, which gave us a method of distinguishing between the different varieties of haemolytic streptococci. This method had not, at that time, been employed in attempts to solve a problem such as ours, but a few simple biochemical tests soon showed that the two varieties were not only different from each other, but both were different from those that cause puerperal fever.

Then began a strange transatlantic collaboration between the two of us, in which she sent me sera and I sent her strains of haemolytic streptococci I had isolated. Nowadays such a proceeding would pose few problems because the aeroplane ensures delivery of parcels within a day or so. But in order to make certain that packages would not be delayed so long that the microbes died before they reached her, I had to add to my other duties by becoming an expert on the sailing dates of transatlantic liners.

It was worth it, because she found that one of the two varieties I had isolated from the pregnant woman was the same as that which causes a disease of cattle called mastitis. Subsequent work has shown that such strains are comparatively common inhabitants of the human vagina. But how or why they get there, no one knows to this day. The other variety was a new discovery. It was one that she had never encountered before. It was later found that it belonged to a group that causes tonsillitis in dogs. Her analysis of the remaining strains showed clearly that, although haemolytic streptococci may be present in the vagina before delivery, they are not capable of producing puerperal fever.[57]

If, then, obstetricians had been wrong in thinking that the haemolytic streptococci causing puerperal fever had been in the birth canal before delivery, where had they come from? This question was answered for us by Dr John Smith of Aberdeen who demonstrated in a masterly piece of work which, in my opinion, has never received the attention it deserves, that they usually come from the nose or throat of one or other of the attendants at the time of delivery.[73] But lest anyone should think that this is an Aberdonian peculiarity, Dora Colebrook showed that Sassenach midwives and obstetricians in London could infect women in very much the same way.[8]

All this suggested ways and means of preventing puerperal

fever caused by haemolytic streptococci. The first was the wearing of a mask. Strange as it may seem even this elementary precaution was unknown at that time. In fact one eminent obstetrician told me that he dare not wear one. His patients might think he was protecting himself from their microbes. The second was the wearing of sterile gloves. This too, was almost unknown, particularly by midwives and general practitioners. One reason was that they were expensive and difficult to sterilize. To get over this difficulty, Colebrook began looking for an antiseptic that would kill streptococci on the bare hands. None of those available were suitable for this purpose.

At this point the Colebrook clan, which was large and widespread, held a get-together somewhere in the vicinity of London, and Colebrook met a distant cousin who was a chemist by profession. Colebrook told him of his problem and he came to the laboratory to see us. He turned out to be an extremely talkative individual, but it emerged that he was on the staff of Messrs Reckitt who, amongst other things, make the blue that is used in laundries. He had ideas about a suitable compound, and in due course it was produced. Related to carbolic acid, it was a chloroxylenol, and much less poisonous.

Unfortunately, it had to be dissolved in an aromatic oil with a very penetrating odour, so penetrating that it attached itself to my clothes and I was asked searching questions when I got home about my activities during the day.

It was what Colebrook wanted, but to make sure that it could kill streptococci on the skin of the hands he carried out a great many experiments in which he smeared his hands with living cultures of these highly virulent organisms and then applied the new antiseptic. He always took a good look at his hands before doing so to see whether there were any cuts or abrasions through which the organisms might penetrate into the deeper tissues to produce infection. He did in fact escape such a catastrophe, but I will never forget the look of horror that came into his eyes when a surgeon told him afterwards that the microbe, if so minded, could apparently penetrate unbroken skin, or at least skin with no visible lesion.

Thus was born the antiseptic we know today as Dettol.

Colebrook was forever singing its praises. So much so that the more cynical of his friends thought he had a pecuniary interest in it. I am quite certain he did not.

With all this, Colebrook now possessed not only the necessary knowledge but some of the means whereby a great many cases of puerperal fever could be prevented. In this he was in his element. For he was a born missionary, impelled by subconscious forces to eradicate disease in human beings. This was no recently acquired trait. Indeed, he had trained to become a medical missionary, but after a spell in Wright's laboratory learning bacteriology, he discovered that Great Britain could provide him with quite enough disease to eradicate. Perhaps this was as well, for in other climates, dealing with less tolerant people, he might have ended his life as a martyr. Even so I have no doubt he had several narrow escapes, for he now proceeded to bully, cajole, wheedle and even order – as the occasion demanded – unwilling obstetric surgeons and even more hide-bound and custom-ridden matrons and midwives to alter their ways and adopt a whole series of what they thought were new-fangled and almost ludicrous innovations which, so he told them, would prevent puerperal fever.

When the Second World War came, he used the same methods to persuade the surgeons to adopt techniques that might prevent infection of wounds and particularly burns. This led him far afield, for after narrowly escaping capture in France following Dunkirk, he made his way to Glasgow. He found the Glaswegians somewhat resistant to the reforms he tried to persuade them to adopt. Perhaps it was because he was a Sassenach, for when he eventually reached the Birmingham Accident Hospital his fellow countrymen were much more receptive. Here he revolutionized the treatment of burns. For all this he was, deservedly, given his F.R.S. in 1945 and Honorary Fellowships of the Royal College of Surgeons and the Royal College of Obstetricians and Gynaecologists.

Even when he retired in 1946 he was by no means idle, and it was mainly by his efforts that a Private Member's Bill was passed by Parliament, which ensured the provision of safeguards on heating appliances in order to lessen the danger of accidents in the home.

This was his *forte:* the use of data obtained in all sorts of ways, including laboratory experiments, to support a particular crusade. And how well equipped he was to use it. The beetling eyebrows, the piercing eyes, the rather cracked voice, and above all the tearing sincerity and fearless honesty of the man, wedded to a remarkable courage that made him oblivious of the consequences of whatever he might say. There were few who remained unconvinced after hearing what Colebrook told them they should do.

I have no doubt that following the work of Dr John Smith, Dora Colebrook, Dr Lancefield and myself, which provided him with the necessary information by the end of 1934, Colebrook did prevent a great deal of puerperal fever in the years that followed. But it is impossible to prove this because, as Prof. L. P. Garrod put it, 'something was brewing in the Rhineland' about that time. The fact that the 'brew' had evidently reached the bottling stage was brought home to me while Colebrook was away on holiday in the summer of 1935. It had always been his custom when away to delegate the handling of his correspondence to me, and on this occasion there arrived a postcard from his friend, Dr Claud Lillingston, who lived in Paris and kept him informed about developments on the Continent. The postcard merely told him that a new compound called Prontosil had been introduced for the treatment of streptococcal infections, and gave the reference to the paper describing it. My reaction was to throw the postcard down to await Colebrook's return, with the thought, 'Another of those damned compounds from Germany with a trade name and of unknown composition that are no use anyway.'

What I thought on this occasion may bring home to those who did not live through this period what bacteriologists thought about chemical compounds for the treatment of bacterial infections. None of us, not even the inhabitants of the Inoculation Department, were as Maurois supposed hostile to them. But we were, time and again, infuriated by the claims put forward by clinicians and commercial firms for compounds that should never have been introduced into medicine at all. Nor was their introduction conducted on a quiet or modest scale. Mercurochrome, to which I have already referred, required no less than 111 pages of a reputable surgical journal to describe its supposed virtues. Sanocrysin and antivirus had required whole books. Nor need anyone think that this sort of thing is extinct. Less than 10 years ago I was present at the coming-out party for a new compound said to prevent colds. It took no more than a glance to see that the evidence in support of it was worthless, and nothing has been heard of it since. But to judge by the amount of alcohol provided for the journalists who attended the party, the drug firm that introduced it cannot have thought so at that time. It was behaviour of this sort that made us all extremely dubious about any new compound.

With this in mind, I doubt whether I would have taken the trouble to go to the Royal Society of Medicine to consult the paper even if the postcard had been addressed to me. But Colebrook on his return, being wiser, consulted the paper in question and made a startling discovery. This was that a German Professor, Gerhard Domagk, who was Director of the Institute of Experimental Pathology attached to the I. G. Farben Industrie at Elberfeld, had evidently discovered that a deep red dye called Prontosil could apparently prevent death of mice infected by haemolytic streptococci. Only one experiment was quoted that showed this, but very remarkable results had been obtained: 12 mice that had received one dose of the drug by stomach tube 1½ hours after an intraperitoneal injection of the organisms survived for 7 days, whereas 13 out of 14 control mice had died within 3 days and the last on the 4th.[20]

This was all very well but there were no references to other experiments of the same nature, and to make it look even more like a fluke the experiment had apparently been carried out on December 20, 1932 whereas the paper had been published on February 15, 1935 in the *Deutsche Medizinische Wochenschrift*. And to make the story even more improbable, it was specifically stated that the compound had no action on streptococci in the test tube.

Two other papers in the same number of the journal described the clinical uses of the compound,[55, 72] and further enquiry showed that others giving rather unsatisfactory reports on cases treated with it or a very similar compound called Streptozon S, had appeared in 1933[42] and 1934.[45] The bacteriological investigations had been carried out so badly that there was even doubt what variety of organisms were causing the infection in some of them.

More details about the history of the compound were given on October 3 by Professor Heinrich Hoerlein, a chemist and Director of the Bayer Laboratories, in a lecture at the Royal Society of Medicine.[52]

Not without difficulty, because the Germans seemed to be unwilling to let him have any Prontosil, Colebrook then began a long series of experiments which showed that, as Domagk had said, the new compound had no direct action on streptococci. He therefore had to do what everyone in the school of Wright hated doing, test the compound in mice. Not because of any dislike of vivisection, but because the current doctrine was that infection of animals by injecting organisms was so artificial a proceeding that any lessons learned as a result would probably not be applicable to naturally acquired human infections. The causation and pathology of such infections were judged to be very different.

On this particular occasion this idea appeared to be justified, because the compound had no action when tested with any of six different strains of haemolytic streptococci all recently isolated from cases with puerperal fever. This almost sounded its death knell, but fortunately Dr G. A. H. Buttle, who had also been studying the compound in the Wellcome Laboratories in Beckenham, appeared on the scene, heralded as was usually his custom, by one of the most stentorian laughs I have ever heard, and told Colebrook that more virulent strains were better indicators of the value of Prontosil. He produced one which was more suitable and, sure enough, Prontosil could cure mice infected by it.

By Christmas, 1935, Colebrook was beginning to satisfy himself about Prontosil. This was fortunate for me, because on January 16, 1936, I pricked myself in the laboratory with a sliver of glass contaminated by haemolytic streptococci and within a day or two it was beginning to be doubtful whether I would survive. By this time I had become a patient in St Mary's and was too ill to protest when Colebrook appeared and gave me Prontosil intravenously and tablets to swallow every few hours. I thereupon became a bright pink in colour and felt so much worse that I began to wonder whether I was dying because of the drug or the microbes. It may well be that Fleming, who had an eye for colour, thought the same, because all he could say to my wife after coming to see me was, 'Hae ye said your prayers?'

My friend Prof. C. A. Pannett, who also has an eye for colour, being a water-colour painter of no mean ability, was more practical in his approach and performed several operations so that I turned the corner in 10 days. I even succeeded in recovering the full use of my hand, an almost unprecedented sequel to infections of this type.

Previous to my tinctorial metamorphosis in mid-January, Colebrook had only treated one or two rather mild cases of puerperal fever. But while I was away regaining my complexion he started to use Prontosil in earnest. This was his great opportunity. Probably knowing more about the disease than anyone else in the world, and having the hospital under his own control, the clinicians having learned that it was best to leave him alone, he proceeded to put Prontosil through its paces.

The first question to be answered was how the drug was to be tested. Should it be on a sound statistical basis with treatment being given only to half the patients, leaving the other half to die (or perhaps, more correctly, 25 per cent of them, as had been the case before Prontosil arrived); should it be given to only the more severely infected; or should it be given to all of them? The first required more courage and hard-heartedness than anyone possessed, the second would inevitably founder on determination of the dividing line between the more and the less serious, so that, like Roux when faced with the same dilemma following the discovery of diphtheria antitoxin, we were left with the third alternative.

Statistically, this was all wrong; but by this time the 'team'; Colebrook, Meave Kenny, Fry and Elizabeth White, had developed a sixth sense which, in Colebrook's case at least, had come to him as a result of all the long years of failure when he had been trying to show that his arsenicals were of some value. Someday, somehow, a statistician may find out how to program hard-won knowledge of this kind for a computer. But this day has not yet arrived and certainly, in 1936, Colebrook and his team could nearly always give an accurate prognosis of what was likely to be the outcome of the illness within a few hours of the arrival of the patient.

And so, depending more on art than on science, they began to treat the patients. I was no more than a spectator but I soon sensed that a change had come. Patients whom we would have given up before now recovered easily, and without the long-drawn-out desperate illness that would previously have been their lot. In consequence, there were only 3 deaths amongst the 38 cases treated during the first 6 months of 1936, and none at all amongst another 26 admitted during the second half of that year. A death rate of only 4·6 per cent for streptococcal infections in the puerperium was unheard of, or as Colebrook himself put it, 'something we had never seen before in ten years' experience of the disease'.

Even so, there were some who doubted; some who thought that, for an unexplained reason, the virulence of the streptococci had suddenly fallen. What is more, they had some justification because patients with puerperal fever were also sent to the North-Western Fever Hospital in Hampstead but had not received Prontosil because the medical officers could not obtain it. Their death rate in the first half of 1936 was only 5·26 per cent. And although there was evidence suggesting that these patients had been less seriously infected than ours, all this made Prof. Topley, the bacteriological pontiff of the country at that time, extremely suspicious of the *bona fides* of Prontosil. If he had had his way, it is improbable that anything further would have been heard of it. For he was a great believer in statistics.

Colebrook and Meave Kenny published their paper in the *Lancet* on June 6, 1936.[13] It was accompanied by an editorial whose writer urged the greatest caution in accepting their results. He had obviously not been one of my visitors at St Mary's earlier in the year.

However improbable the story may have seemed in the

summer of 1935 when I read Dr Lillingston's postcard, it was fact by the time the Second International Congress of Microbiology met in London in July 1936.

Amongst the visitors were Dr and Mrs Tréfouël from the Pasteur Institute in Paris, who came down to Queen Charlotte's to see us. They had made a most important discovery to which I will refer in more detail in the following chapter. This was that the bright pink colour I had acquired when I was given Prontosil in January had been unnecessary, and was not an essential part of the treatment. What had cured me was only half the Prontosil molecule, a colourless compound called sulphanilamide. And shortly before their visit our biochemist Albert Fuller had forged the last link in the chain of experiments that proved this, by finding sulphanilamide in the urine of patients being treated with Prontosil.[44] As a result of all this, sulphanilamide was soon to replace Prontosil for the treatment of infections.

At the time of their arrival, very few of the other visitors to the Congress knew of the revolution that was about to start. News travelled slowly in those days. But the morning of July 28 was devoted to a session on the streptococci, under the chairmanship of the great Hans Zinsser of *Rats, Lice and History* fame, and most of the papers by Dr G. J. Hucker, Dr F. Griffith, Dr A. W. Stableforth, Dr C. A. Green and myself dealt with the classification of these organisms; a dull subject if ever there was one. Then came a paper by Perrin Long of the Johns Hopkins Hospital, describing experiments with antisera produced in rabbits for the treatment of infections. The mere fact that he had produced them, and that if they had ever come into use would have been fantastically expensive, was in a sense a little light relief. Another series of dull papers followed, so dull I cannot even remember their authors. Last of all came Colebrook. He was to have talked about anaerobic streptococci but explained that he would rather tell them about Prontosil. Although he described the cures at Queen Charlotte's and his sincerity was so obvious that they all believed him, there was no ovation. After all, we had been at it all the morning, the room was hot and we wanted lunch.

During the afternoon I met Perrin Long and asked him what

he proposed to do with all the antistreptococcal sera he had been making now that we had Prontosil. He did not know what I was talking about, but it transpired that he had left the meeting after his own paper to see Howard Brown, also of Baltimore, whose monograph on haemolysis by the streptococci is a bacteriological classic. Brown had been 'incarcerated' in University College Hospital because he had forgotten that we drive on the left-hand side of the road and a taxi had forcibly reminded him of the fact. For this reason Perrin Long had not heard Colebrook's paper, nor did he know that I owed my life to Prontosil.

Without waiting to enquire further, he straightaway cancelled his projected trip on the Continent, obtained a booking on the next boat home, cabled the pharmacist at Johns Hopkins Hospital to beg, borrow or steal some Prontosil and sulphanilamide, introduced my wife and me to Bourbon whisky at the English Speaking Union that evening, and returned to America to find practically no Prontosil available and the only sulphanilamide in existence in the New World being made specially for him by the Jackson Laboratory of the DuPont Company. Despite these hindrances he succeeded, with Dr Eleanor Bliss, in confirming that these drugs could cure infected mice. They then cured a child with erysipelas, a woman with puerperal fever, and several others with quinsy and otitis media, reported these results at a meeting of the Southern Medical Association in November, and published them in the *Journal of the American Medical Association* on January 2, 1937.

And so, without benefit of blind trials, Latin squares, computers and other statistical devices and, in fact, in face of what statistical evidence there was, the chemotherapy of bacterial infections was born.

Nevertheless, the new-born baby was very different from the one that had been expected. Even the most optimistic of bacteriologists had thought that any compound capable of curing a bacterial infection would be, fundamentally, an antiseptic in being a general protoplasmic poison that acted by coagulating the proteins in the bacterial cell. Its only difference from carbolic acid or mercury perchloride, for example, being that it would be rather less poisonous for the cells of the patient than for those of the microbe. Because of this, even a slight overdose would almost inevitably be fatal. It would also have to be administered by intravenous injection and, because of its inherent poisonous properties, more or less serious damage to important organs such as the kidneys, liver and even the brain could be anticipated.

When Prontosil and the other sulphonamides eventually appeared, all these ideas went by the board. Not only were they apparently harmless but they could even be taken by the mouth.

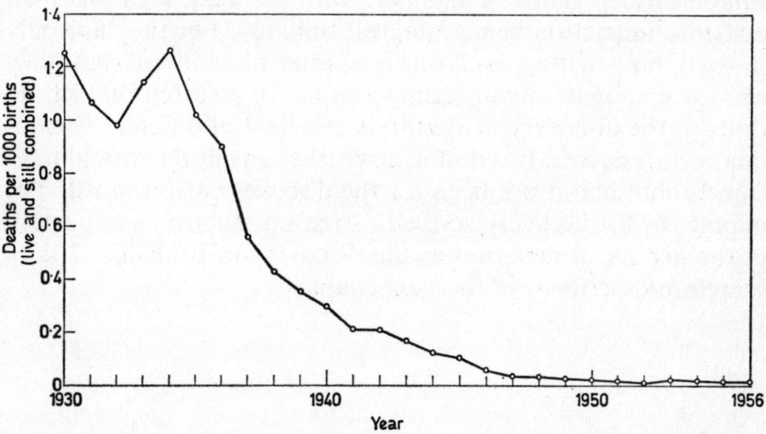

Fig. 2. Deaths from puerperal fever in England and Wales, showing the fall following the introduction of the sulphonamides and penicillin.

Nor did their mode of action bear any resemblance to the crudity of the antiseptics. All that they could, or apparently needed to do, was to interfere with the growth and reproduction of the microbes. They need not even go so far as to kill them, for unless a microbe can go through the various phases of its life cycle in due order and without interference, it becomes a spent force in so far as the production of infection is concerned.

Although all the modern chemotherapeutic agents act in this way, the processes by which the microbes are rendered impotent vary with the agent concerned. The details do not matter but they generally involve the microbe stealing the enzymes by which the microbe normally lives, grows and reproduces itself. As a result, its digestive system may be upset, or the manner in which the bacterial tissues are constructed are put out of gear. But the eventual outcome, however it is brought about, is such disorganization of the life cycle of the microbe that it ceases to be a menace to its natural host.

No one, so far as I know, had prophesied that these substances would act so differently from the antiseptics or in so comparatively gentle a manner. But the new ideas had an immense impact on bacteriological thinking. For they not only showed how wrong had our previous ideas been, but they opened up apparently unending avenues of research that led, in time, to the discovery or synthesis of a host of different chemotherapeutic agents. It is doubtful whether any of this would have come about had it not been for the discovery of Prontosil. The manner of its discovery is, for this reason, almost as important in the history of mankind as the discovery of penicillin. I shall therefore describe it in the next chapter.

Chapter 8

Molecules and Microbes

It is, I think, usually assumed that scientists resemble computers in being totally devoid of emotion, humour, and aesthetic feeling who spend their lives churning out facts and figures that are generally incomprehensible to anyone but themselves. The early history of penicillin shows how far from the truth this form of generalization can be. So was that of the sulphonamides. Their early history was almost as long, equally tortuous and beset by human frailty. It is for this reason that I propose to describe it in some detail.

Prontosil was discovered in the research laboratories of the I.G. Farben Industrie at Elberfeld in the Ruhr, not far from Düsseldorf. This was an enormous organization, specializing in the manufacture of chemical compounds of all kinds. One of its activities was the production of dyestuffs for use in the textile industry. Pharmaceutical substances seem to have been a relatively minor part of their activities.

Although Prontosil was the result of the work of a team, most of the credit must go to Gerhard Domagk. Born in 1895, he qualified in medicine in 1921, following service as a grenadier in the First World War. After acting as assistant to Hoppe Seyler, the biochemist, he was appointed, at the early age of 32, Director of research in experimental pathology and bacteriology in the Institute attached to the I.G. Farben works at Elberfeld. He remained there for the rest of his life, dying in 1964.

As well as the discovery of Prontosil, he was largely responsible for the introduction into medicine of a series of antiseptics known as the quaternary ammonium compounds. Zephiran and Cetrimide are examples. He also showed that a number of sulphur-containing compounds, the thiosemicarbazones, could be used for the treatment of patients with tuberculosis. Towards the end of his life, he turned his attention to the chemotherapy of cancer. He was, therefore, a bacteriologist of very considerable distinction, was made F.R.S. in 1959 and was given the Nobel Prize for Medicine in 1939.

I met him only once, when he lectured – in remarkably good English – at St Mary's after the war. By all accounts, he was a charming and cultured man.[12]

His discovery of Prontosil was largely due to the fact that he was the bacteriologist in a co-operative effort in which chemists played a considerable part. The method was very similar to that employed by Ehrlich which resulted in the discovery of 606, or Arsphenamine, for the treatment of syphilis. This was, as a chemist has put it, 'patient research which involved finding a suitable therapeutic nucleus and by proper substitution on this, enhancing its effect to the maximum',[64] but which, for those unacquainted with chemical jargon, may be translated as, 'first find a compound that looks promising and then tinker with it until something better emerges'.

Even so, it is doubtful whether Prontosil would have been discovered had it not been for the fact that animal tests were employed for the evaluation of any new compounds. This had been essential in Erhlich's researches because he was working with trypanosomes and, later, spirochaetes. Neither can be cultivated in the bacteriological media of the laboratory, so that animals had to be used to provide living organisms for his tests and to detect whether or not they had survived contact with the compounds he was using. When, however, the Germans were searching for substances that might be used for the treatment of bacterial infections, it seemed at first that since these organisms multiply in bacteriological media in the test tube, the expensive and time-consuming animal tests might, in the preliminary stages at least, be dispensed with.

This was the prevailing doctrine at that time; it being assumed that any compound that had no action on bacteria in the test tube was unlikely to be of much value in the living body. But in the course of their work, they observed that compounds might have no action on bacteria *in vitro*, but could, in spite of this, kill them in the body of an experimental animal. Such compounds were referred to as 'true chemotherapeutic substances' in order, I suppose, to distinguish them from the antiseptics that, being general protoplasmic poisons, can kill them under all circumstances.

How such a compound acted as a successful chemotherapeutic substance did not seem to matter, or at any rate could be left out of account, until time was available to find out.

Domagk and his fellow workers accordingly resolved to rely on animal tests for the evaluation of their compounds. This change in thinking and procedure was of very considerable importance if only because it resulted in the discovery of Prontosil.

The first step that led to it seems to have been nothing more than the 'screening' of every new compound produced by the industrial empire that employed Domagk, or which someone thought might bear investigation. The objective was no more than to find out whether it had any activity at all. I think it must have been this procedure that Wright saw when he visited Elberfeld and regaled us at tea with the story that he had been shown enormous laboratories in which they did nothing but take compound after compound and test its ability to deal with infections in animals caused by a variety of organisms. Blind groping in the dark in this way was so utterly foreign to someone of Wright's temperament that he looked on it as a form of sacrilege. To him, the only method was to think the thing out in the privacy of one's study and then do the experiment to prove the theory.

However unintellectual the method may have been it was better than nothing, and in the end paid dividends. The first substance to be detected in this way was a gold compound. But no matter what was done to the molecule, it was too toxic to be of any use. The same applied to a compound of arsenic and antimony and still other compounds containing tin.[21] They then turned their attention to the azo-dyes. These are compounds whose molecules have a peculiar architecture to which I will presently refer. They possess one great merit in that they do not kill the animals even though they stain the tissues. Moreover they can kill microbes, and sometimes in high dilution. But in spite of this, those that they tested were unable to cure infected animals. Even when the molecules were modified in one way or another, the best that could be done was to render them capable of killing bacteria in the test tube in higher dilution than did the parent dye. But this did not convert them into useful chemotherapeutic agents.

While this was in progress, the chemists responsible for the production of dyes for use in the textile industry had been synthesizing another series of azo-dyes. This was an outcome of work carried out many years previously by the I.G. Farben chemists, Hoerlein, Dressel and Kothe. They had found that, in technical language, if a sulphamyl group (H_2NSO_2) was introduced into the azo-dye molecule in the *para* position relative to the N-linkage, it became a much better dye when used for protein materials such as wool or silk. Such a dye penetrated so deeply and remained so firmly fixed to the fibres that textiles dyed with it were better able to resist the harmful effects of washing, fulling and exposure to light.

Apparently by pure chance, a compound of this nature seems to have reached Domagk who found that it possessed definite ability to cure infection of mice by haemolytic streptococci. This was what would nowadays be called the breakthrough, or, as Hoerlein put it when he spoke at the Royal Society of Medicine in October 1935, 'The observation of Domagk on the action of one of these dyes on streptococci directed our subsequent work into a new channel. Numerous new azo-dyes containing sulphonamide were prepared but the test object was no longer the wool fibre but the mouse infected with streptococci.' And as a result, 'Mietzsch and Klarer in close collaboration with Domagk preparaed a large number of compounds of great activity whose effects on streptococcal infections excelled all those previously observed in animal experiments'.[52]

In view of what is to follow, we must consider, as far as possible, in non-technical language, exactly what they had done.

They had taken a dye such as chrysoidin which is a rather uninteresting orange-yellow in colour and whose structural formula is as follows:

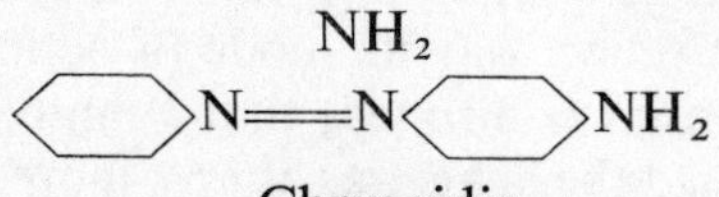

Chrysoidin

They had then added what is known as a sulphamyl group, that is to say one atom of nitrogen (N), one of sulphur (S) and two each of hydrogen (H) and oxygen (O), expressed as H_2NSO_2 to the western end of the molecule to produce a new dye called sulphamido-chrysoidin.

This procedure not only gave the new compound a rich red ruby colour but rendered it capable of curing bacterial infections in mice. Its formula is as follows:

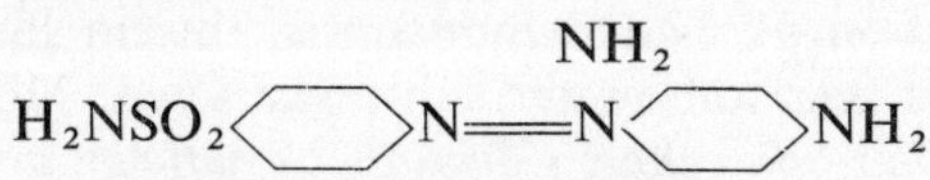

Sulphamido-chrysoidin

It was the behaviour of this dye, given the trade name Prontosil, later changed to Prontosil rubrum that was the subject of the paper by Domagk, published on February 15, 1935, that led, as I have described in the preceding chapter, to the introduction of the sulphonamides into medicine.

One of the first to appreciate the importance of this discovery seems to have been Constantin Levaditi, a Rumanian working in Paris. Probably doubting the whole story like the rest of us, he asked I.G. Farben for samples of the new drug. They refused and again when he asked them a second time. This did not deter him for he invoked the aid of Prof. E. Fourneau, who was Chief of the Laboratory of Therapeutic Chemistry in the Pasteur Institute. In a few weeks Dr A. Girard, a member of his staff, produced a bottle of red crystals closely resembling Prontosil. He had used the patent specification to synthesize them. Although their composition was subsequently found to be slightly different, they too, as Levaditi and his assistant Vaisman soon found, could cure infections in mice. This new compound was called Rubiazol.[58]

Having something comparable to Prontosil with which to work, the next question was its mode of action. Domagk had said, and it was soon confirmed, that Prontosil could not kill microbes in the test tube. This was almost more remarkable than its ability to cure infections. Many years previously Paul Ehrlich, the father of chemotherapy, had enunciated the doctrine, and in order to make it more impressive had put it into Latin, that '*Corpora non agunt, nisi fixatur*', but here was something that might possibly fix itself to the microbes but did not kill them. Antiseptics could do so, and so did the arsenicals. But this one was very abnormal.

On the other hand, whatever might be the mechanism by which Prontosil cured infections, the microbes certainly disappeared from the peritoneum of a mouse while it was under treatment. Domagk had demonstrated this in his paper. But he gave no clue as to how the substance acted. All he could say was that it was '*ein echtes Chemotherapeuticum nur in lebenden Organismus*', which does no more than state the obvious. But he did go so far as to say that it did not act by stimulating the reticulo-endothelial system to unusual activity. This was one way of expressing a concept current at that time which was usually referred to as non-specific immunization. It implied that infections might be cured by the injection of compounds having no direct action on the microbes but which could, in some undefined way, boost the anti-bacterial mechanisms to such unusual activity that they, not the compound itself, cured the infection. It has still to be proved that this is possible.

Nothing more than this was known when Dr and Mrs Tréfouël, with Drs Nitti and Bovet of the Pasteur Institute, took up the problem. Since the work they did was of great importance, it will be necessary to describe it in some detail. Much depends on the structural formula of Prontosil. I shall therefore describe it as far as possible in non-technical language.

The formula of Prontosil is as follows, N denoting one atom of nitrogen, S of sulphur, O of oxygen, and H of hydrogen:

Prontosil rubrum 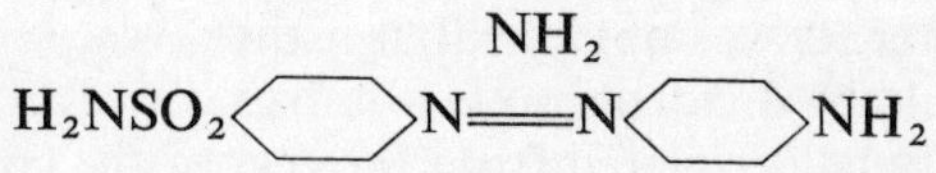

It will be observed that it consists of two hexagons or benzene rings joined end to end. That on the left or western end is by far the most important and, to employ a geographical analogy, can be represented by Devon and Cornwall from Land's End to Exeter. Here, at the eastern end of this hexagon, the two nitrogen atoms can be represented by the two halves of the city on each side of the river Exe and the double bond uniting them is the road and railway bridges crossing the river. If we ignore the other roads and railways to the north of Exeter, these bridges become the only link between Devon and Cornwall and the rest of England. Let us also assume that the remaining angles on this hexagon are capes, those on its southern side being The Lizard and Start Point; those on the northern side Trevose Head and Hartland Point.

The eastern hexagon is much less important and can be represented by as much of the neighbouring counties as is necessary for the compound under discussion.

Up to this point, there has been no mention of the Scilly Isles. They will do duty for the single atoms of sulphur and nitrogen and the two atoms of hydrogen and oxygen that constitute the sulphamyl group.

Let us now return to Paris and the Pasteur Institute with Dr Tréfouël and his colleagues looking at the map. One of the first features that must have attracted their attention was the position of the Scilly Isles. They were at Land's End. But because the only point on a benzene ring to which anything can be attached is one of the angles, the Scillies might have been attached to The Lizard or Start Point. And, since geographical engineering is not beyond the capacity of the modern chemist, they tried moving them to these headlands. But this procedure virtually annihilated the chemotherapeutic activity of the molecule. The Scillies had to be at Land's End or, in technical language, the sulphamyl group had to be in the *para* position relative to the N-linkage and not in the *ortho* or *meta* positions.

They would then have turned their attention to the bridges at

Exeter. It was obvious that if they were blown up, the molecule would be divided into two halves with Devon, Cornwall and the Scilly Isles isolated from the rest of the country. This would be an easier operation to perform in the living body than at Exeter because all that would be required would be reduction, that is to say, the addition of two hydrogen atoms by means of enzymes that are always present in the living body. In this way, Prontosil would become two separate molecules, one being sulphanilamide and the other tri-amino-benzene as follows:

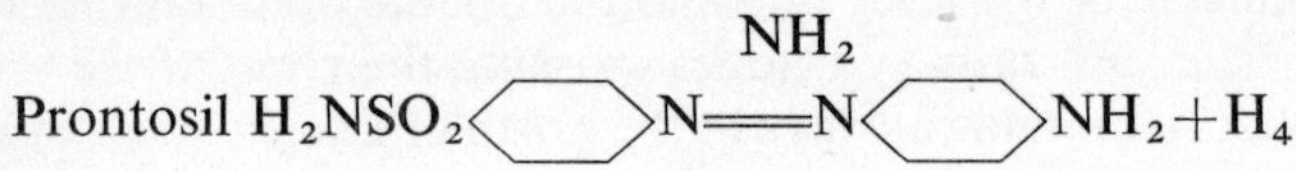

to give

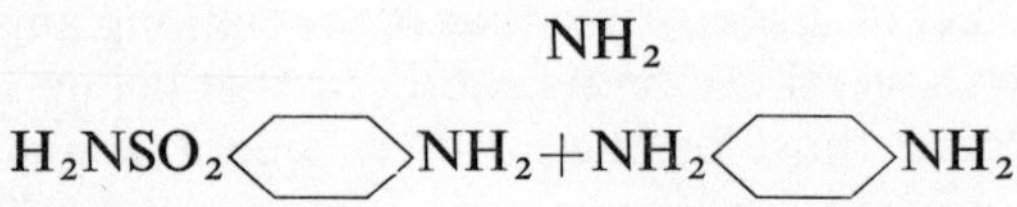

Sulphanilamide Tri-amino-benzene

Having 'blown the bridges' the next question was: Which of the two halves acted as the chemotherapeutic agent? The clue to this was provided by work carried out by Dr Michael Heidelberger of New York, another visitor to the Congress in 1936, who came to my house in order, with my wife and a friend who was a violinist, to play Brahms horn trios he had transposed for his clarinet. But long before this, in collaboration with Dr W. A. Jacobs in 1919, he had shown that sulphanilamide coupled with a derivative of quinine could kill microbes in the test tube. Although the chemotherapeutic potentialities of the compound were never tested, this suggested that sulphanilamide might have properties not hitherto suspected.

The French workers accordingly prepared a compound which they called 1162F whose structural formula was as follows:

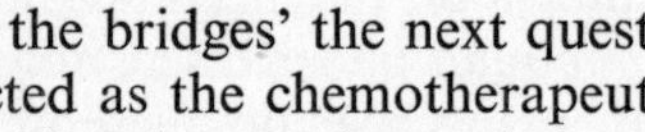

This compound was then used for the treatment of mice and rabbits infected by haemolytic streptococci. It acted in the same way as did Prontosil or Rubiazol. It prevented or cured infection. Since this compound closely resembled the sulphanilamide that would be released if the Prontosil molecule was split at the double bond, the conclusion was warranted that it was the liberation of sulphanilamide that enabled Prontosil to cure infections.

Dr Tréfouël and his colleagues communicated their results to the Society for Biology at their meeting on November 23, 1935, so that the secret of Prontosil's mode of action had already been uncovered within 9 months of Domagk's paper.[74] But for some unknown reason they never proved that liberation of free sulphanilamide did actually occur. This was left for my friend Dr Albert Fuller to demonstrate in the summer of 1936, when he found that it was being excreted by the kidneys of patients under treatment with Prontosil.[44]

If further proof were needed that it was the liberation of sulphanilamide that enabled Prontosil to act as a chemotherapeutic agent, it was also found that, unlike Prontosil, it could act directly on the microbes. Ehrlich had been proved right after all. The real chemotherapeutic agent was sulphanilamide and it did act as Ehrlich required. It did fix itself to the microbes and deal with them. But only after it had been freed from the rest of the molecule by rupture of the double bond. Devon and Cornwall alone, so long as they had the Scilly Isles at Land's End, were quite capable of dealing with the invaders. The rest of Britain was no more than an encumbrance.

These discoveries were of the very greatest importance because they pointed the way to the synthesis of new compounds that would deal with other microbes besides streptococci, meningococci and gonococci, the microbial species for which sulphanilamide was of most value. But it was soon found that there were limits as to what could be done with the molecule. Little, for example, was gained by altering its eastern end. Except for a few compounds where a county or two were added on the other side of the bridges at Exeter, that end of the molecule was best left alone.

The really important part was the western end and particularly the Scillies. They had to be at Land's End, as I have already pointed out, but even their constituent atoms had to be left alone. In fact, all that was possible was replacement of one of the hydrogen atoms by something else. In the process, quite large amounts of land were sometimes required. So much so that for some compounds, it was necessary to bring about a re-emergence of the lost land of Lionesse from beneath the waves round the Scilly Islands. Our old friend Dr Ewins was one of the first to produce the submarine explosion required for this purpose and brought up almost a whole county with no less than six capes (in technical language, a pyridine nucleus) to produce sulphapyridine. Because of this, it was of great value for the treatment of pneumonia caused by the pneumococcus. Not very long afterwards, in 1943, he was given his F.R.S. at the same time as Fleming.

Sulphapyridine

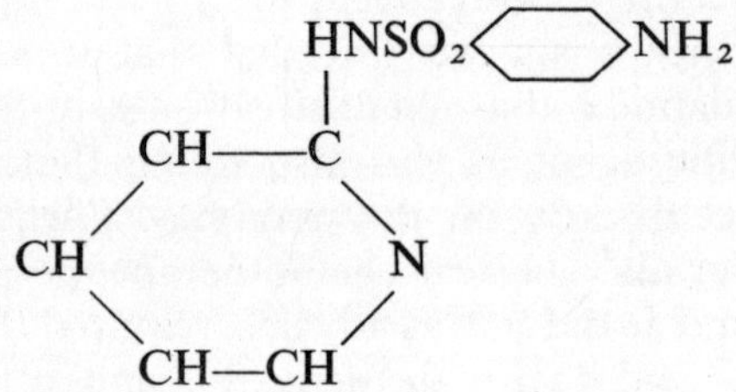

Another compound was sulphathiazole which had to make do with only five capes but in spite of this could deal with staphylococci that generally resisted treatment by the compounds already mentioned.

Sulphathiazole

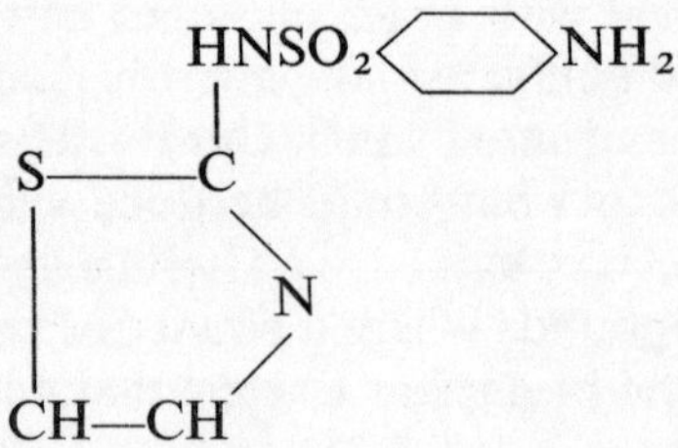

Other compounds were, territorially, much less ambitious. One was sulphaguanidine, still used by our doctor when he gives us something when we go abroad and fear the stomach upsets that so frequently spoil our holidays in hot climates. It is quite content with no more than a few islands.

Sulphaguanidine

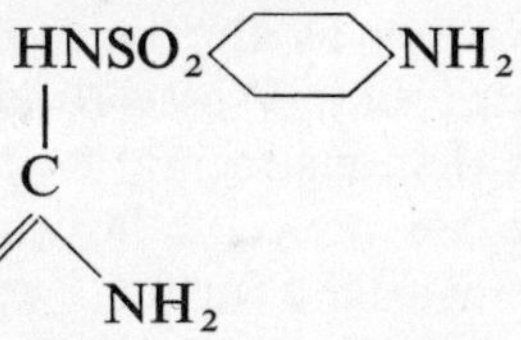

Up to this point, the story of the sulphonamides has been relatively simple and straightforward. But soon after Prontosil appeared, questions began to be asked. Why was it that Domagk's solitary mouse experiment had been dated December 20, 1932, but the paper describing so sensational a discovery was not published until February 1935, 2 years and 3 months later? Why had the Germans been evidently so unwilling to allow samples of the new drug to go abroad for testing? Levaditi had asked twice and been refused each time; Sir Henry Dale could not obtain samples for testing by the Therapeutic Trials Committee in the spring of 1935; and even in the autumn of that year, Colebrook had difficulty in getting supplies.

The official reason was given by Hoerlein in 1937, in a paper read to the British Association and reported in *The Practitioner* in the following words: 'The first German patent for Prontosil (No. 607,537) is dated Christmas Day, 1932. Example I of the patent gives details of the manufacture of a red dyestuff (today known as Prontosil rubrum) by diazotising *para*-amino-phenyl-sulphonamide (nowadays known as Prontosil album) and combining the diazo compound with *meta*-phenylene-diamine. The results obtained with these and similar compounds seemed, however, too good to be true, so that before publishing them several years were devoted to intensive clinical and experimental work. This explains why Domagk, the Director of the experimental pathological laboratory, delayed publishing the results of the chemotherapeutic action of Prontosil in experimental infections in mice and rabbits until February, 1935.'[53]

Taken at its face value, this seems perfectly reasonable. Domagk was merely being more cautious than is usual. But unfortunately Hoerlein did not mention what they were really doing, what their problems were or how they solved them. Nor is Domagk's paper at all helpful. It does, it is true, describe such fundamental matters as the lack of toxicity of Prontosil, its action on the heart, blood vessels and muscles, but it quotes only one experiment demonstrating its ability to cure infections in mice, and there are none of the variations on this theme that would be expected after a further 2 years work. And although the effect of the compound on infections in rabbits is also alluded to, the information is extremely scanty.

Anyone acquainted with the testing of new compounds would know that most, if not all the work described in the paper, must have been completed soon after the discovery and certainly before Prontosil was used for the treatment of human patients. Nor were the long term investigations before a new compound can be used, now required since the thalidomide tragedy, even thought of at that time.

It is, however, possible that Domagk may have had more difficulties than he was prepared to admit. He may, for example, have found, as did Colebrook, that it is only when highly virulent and therefore somewhat unusual strains of streptococci are employed that it is possible to demonstrate the curative action of the drug in animals. As a result, he may have been led astray into thinking that only certain types of these organisms are susceptible and this would have taken time to elucidate. But no mention of this is made in the paper.

A second possibility is that it may have been difficult to obtain a sufficient number of well authenticated case reports. But treatment of patients evidently began quite early. The first was in 1933, because a Dr Foerster reported at the monthly meeting of the Düsseldorf Dermatological Society in May 1933 that he had cured a 10-month-old boy suffering from staphylococcal septicaemia with Prontosil soluble.[42] Another report was published in 1934 by a Dr Grutz,[45] and accompanying, or soon after Domagk's paper, there were several.[55, 72] Indeed, it came out in the discussion following Hoerlein's paper in October 1935, that as many as 1,500 cases had been treated in Germany by that time. What is more, Colebrook obtained all the information he required in 6 months at Queen Charlotte's Hospital. It is therefore difficult to believe that there was any lack of clinical material.

It is, however, possible to interpret Hoerlein's excuses in another way. The Germans were, as he said, carrying out intensive experimental work. But this did not concern Prontosil. It was a consequence of the fact that both Hoerlein and Domagk were working for a large industrial concern which was neither a seat of learning, an independent research institute or a charitable organization. It had its shareholders to consider. Practically every new compound was, accordingly, patented so that its subsequent manufacture and sales could be controlled by them. Prontosil was no exception. Had the whole of the Prontosil molecule been required for treatment their profits would have been very large indeed. But it was not; sulphanilamide alone was quite as effective. What is more, it could not be patented. It had been synthesized long before, in Vienna in 1908, by Paul Gelmo as part of the work for his doctor's thesis and who, incidentally, was found eking out a precarious existence after the war in Vienna as an analytical chemist for a firm of printing ink manufacturers.

It is very difficult to believe that the Germans did not become aware of all this and its commercial implications quite early in the proceedings. And certainly there are four very good reasons to suggest this.

The first is that before the end of 1932 they had found not one, but three compounds that were chemotherapeutically active. They were as follows:

1. Probably the first to be discovered, this was not given a name but which I will call the Precursor of Prontosil. It was evidently synthesized in 1931 because it was patented on November 7 of that year. It was not used for the treatment of patients.
2. Prontosil rubrum was probably discovered in 1932, the patent being applied for at Christmas that year but not finally granted until January 2, 1935. This is the compound to which I have so far confined my discussion.

3. This compound was at first called Streptozon S, but because it is more soluble than the foregoing was eventually called Prontosil soluble. It must have been discovered before the end of 1932, because it was this compound that was used by Dr Foerster in May 1933, for the treatment of a patient.

Secondly, to anyone acquainted with the connection between the chemical constitution of compounds and their chemotherapeutic activity, it would be an almost foregone conclusion that all three compounds had something in common. What this was is immediately apparent when their structural formulae are set out as follows:

Precursor of Prontosil

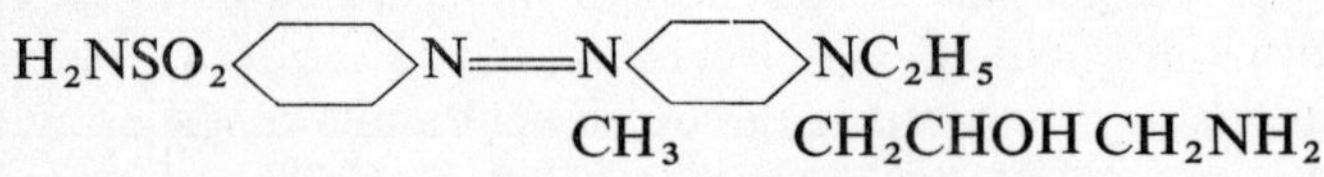

Prontosil rubrum

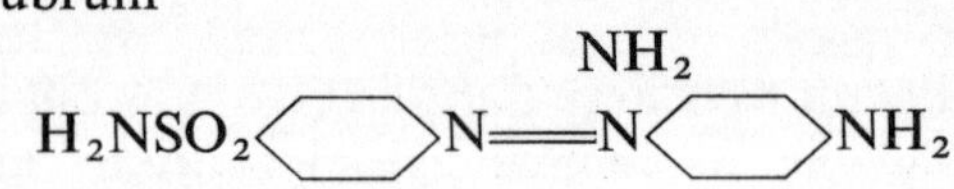

Prontosil soluble or Streptozon S

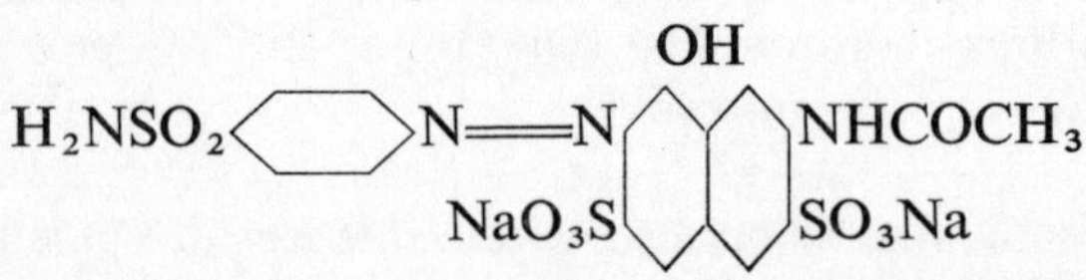

The common factor in all three compounds is the sulphamyl group at the western end of a benzene ring connected to another benzene ring by a double bond.

The third reason why the Germans should have suspected sulphanilamide was suggested to me by Dr Fuller, who pointed out that in the process of synthesizing these compounds the chemist actually starts by taking a bottle labelled sulphanilamide.[50] Some of it is then diazotized by the classical method which involves its treatment with nitrous and hydrochloric acids. All that this causes is, fundamentally, the construction of the double bond uniting the two atoms of nitrogen at the eastern end of the molecule.

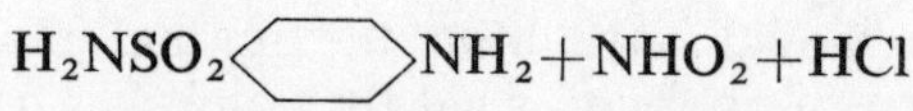

Sulphanilamide Nitrous acid Hydrochloric acid

to give

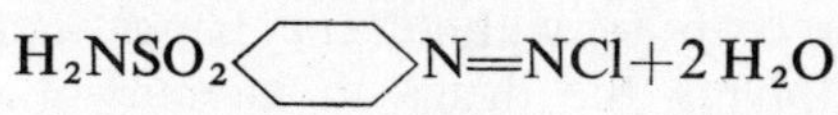

Once the double bond is in position the next step is to couple it to an amine. When Prontosil rubrum is being produced, the amine employed is *meta*-phenylene-diamine. The resulting compound is called sulphamido-chrysoidin, the chemical name for Prontosil rubrum.

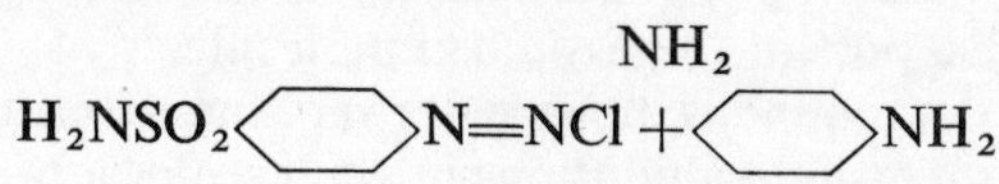

Meta-phenylene-diamine

to give

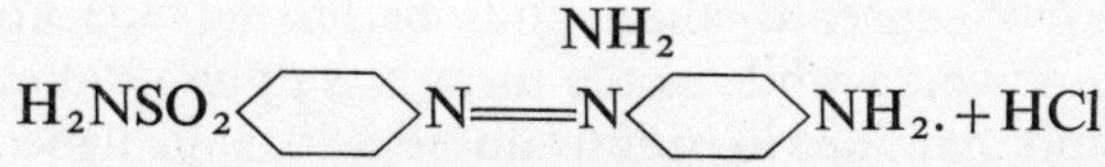

Prontosil rubrum

The fourth and last reason is that, being chemists, they must have known that as a result of simple reduction of any of these compounds in the living body, the double bond could be broken to release sulphanilamide as a free molecule into the circulating blood in the way I have already illustrated.

Thus, with three compounds having the same type of activity as chemotherapeutic agents, their structural formulae all having a sulphamyl-group, their synthesis starting with sulphanilamide and the probability that sulphanilamide would be released by a comparatively simple process in the body, it is difficult to believe that the Germans had not discovered for themselves that sulphanilamide was the real chemotherapeutic agent. And since all three compounds had been synthesized before the end of 1932, it is probable that they may have realized this by that time. If, therefore, Domagk's paper had been published shortly afterwards, which would have been the normal procedure, someone might have soon found what they already knew, that sulphanilamide could act as well as Prontosil.

What then were they to do? The most obvious answer to this question would have been to withold the paper and create difficulties about supplying the drugs to anyone other than clinicians. In other words they played for time. Time in which to attempt the synthesis of compounds having much the same formulae but sufficiently different from sulphanilamide to be capable of protection by patents. With luck, they might even find one that acted on other organisms besides streptococci. This, of course, is exactly what every other pharmaceutical firm attempted to do following the demonstration that sulphanilamide was the active part of the Prontosil molecule.

Finding such a compound is, however, a very time-consuming business because even slight alterations in what seems a promising molecule can render it almost inert. It was for this reason that it took Dr Ewins the best part of 3 years and the testing of no less than 692 separate compounds before he was able to evolve anything worth while in the form of sulphapyridine, the first of the sulphonamides to be introduced into clinical medicine after sulphanilamide.

If this is what the Germans had been doing, it is not surprising that Domagk's paper was delayed so long and that even after its publication they were so unwilling to allow supplies of Prontosil to go to other scientists. But all this playing for time was to no avail. The only sulphonamide they succeeded in producing was Uliron which was not sufficiently different from any of the others to have been worth the trouble.

Assuming that this was the reason for the delay, Domagk does not emerge with very much credit. But, as I have said, he was not a free agent. He had to do as he was told. Nevertheless, the fact remains that his was one of the most important medical discoveries that has ever been made, for it not only enabled us to treat and cure a whole series of very serious forms of infection but, of even greater importance, it showed us how wrong had been our ideas about how a successful chemotherapeutic agent was likely to act. As a consequence of this, penicillin began to be thought of as a possible alternative. But let there be no doubt about it, without the sulphonamides to show the way, it is improbable that penicillin would have emerged from its obscurity.

Chapter 9

Penicillin Proves Itself

Soon after the value of Prontosil had become obvious, it became equally obvious that my days at Queen Charlotte's were numbered. Not only had ways and means been found for preventing puerperal fever, but its cure was also imminent. I had not gone so far as to talk myself out of a job but others had, in a sense, done it for me. The disease I had been hired to study, prevent and cure, seemed likely to disappear or, at least, become less deadly.

Nevertheless, although none of us knew it, the introduction of the sulphonamides led, eventually, to the third phase in the development of penicillin; the demonstration of its value and its manufacture in quantity. Much of this phase I was able to witness rather more closely than most people. How this came about and what I saw of the process may be worth recounting.

My being able to do so was largely due to the fact that ever since I had qualified I had never had secure employment. But I was now married, 36 years old, and for 10 years had had to do the best I could on yearly grants from the Medical Research Council, whose renewal had never been sufficiently certain to avert a great deal of emotion about the time they came up for consideration. But because of this uncertainty I had no prospect of a pension, I dare not buy a house, and it even seemed unwise to start a family.

I had, it is true, learned the rudiments of my profession and had even made a few contributions to knowledge. At all events, others seemed to have thought so because the British Medical Association had given me the Catherine Bishop Harman Prize in

1928, and the Royal Society of Medicine the Nicholls Prize in 1933 which I shared with Dr John Smith. But in spite of this eminence no one seemed disposed to ask for my services. Nor, for that matter were there jobs available. We were in the midst of a severe depression, and what posts there were seemed to be occupied by middle-aged men likely to last a very long time.

Much of the doubt about my future was due to the simple fact that in my desire to make research a whole-time occupation I was ahead of my time. The many opportunities that are now available did not then exist. In fact I think it would be true to say that, until the Second World War, medical research was generally considered unlikely to be of much use to anyone other than the writers of textbooks, and examiners in search of material with which to stump otherwise well-informed candidates at examinations. Its prosecution was, in a sense, a luxury that did not need much support or encouragement, and viewed in the same light as indulgence in such expensive pursuits as salmon fishing or the collection of old masters: something that was best left to those who were financially well enough endowed to afford it, or who were prepared to give up almost everything else in order to prosecute what many regarded as no more than a hobby.

In the circumstances it is perhaps surprising that so much was actually done. But a great deal of it was by men who had taken the precaution to inherit, marry or make sufficient money to enable them to give most of their time to medical research no matter what the state of the employment market might be. Louis Cobbett was, perhaps, the best example. Financially independent, a bachelor, and inhabiting an enormous house in Adams Road where he was looked after by his sister, he did a great deal of important research on diphtheria and tuberculosis in the Pathology Department of Cambridge University. Whatever salary he received – and it cannot have been much – was probably used to pay his gardener. Another such person was Sir Thomas Lewis, the virtual founder of what we know as clinical science. He was a member of a wealthy South Wales coal-owning family but I doubt whether he really needed the salary he received from the Medical Research Council.

Almost equally fortunate were those who acquired wealth by marriage. My own chief Colebrook was one of them. His salary would never have permitted him to buy almost overnight, and without haggling, a large house on Chiswick Mall, build a bungalow in several acres of garden at Farnham Royal and invariably take two very expensive holidays every year. His wife too, became a Governor of the Old Vic at a time when financial as well as moral support was probably required by Lillian Baylis.

Few deliberately set out to make enough money to enable them to do research later in life as did Schliemann the archaeologist. But some came near to it. One such was Dr T. Lumsden who gave up a medical practice while still middle-aged, migrated to the London Hospital and became one of the pioneers of tissue culture for the study of cancer.

Those like myself who had omitted to provide for themselves in this way could, of course, hope for one of the permanent, reasonably well-paid posts in university teaching departments or in the laboratories of such bodies as the Medical Research Council, the Lister Institute, the Imperial Cancer Research Fund and similar laboratories in some of the provincial cities. But anyone who deliberately set out to do research in the hope of getting one was generally considered to be slightly off balance. He might land such a post but the chances were that he would not.

The only other alternative was to make research a spare time occupation or hobby while the necessary bread and butter was earned in some other way. One of the most extreme examples of this was J. E. Barnard. He owned the family hat shop in Jermyn Street but spent most of his spare time at the Hampstead laboratories of the Medical Research Council where he built microscopes to study viruses long before the electron microscope was invented. For those with a medical qualification the usual procedure was for the aspirant to become a pathologist to a hospital. This not only gave him the wherewithal to live in return for the work he did during the day, but the facilities for the research he did during the evenings and at the week-ends. Dedication to such an extent was, admittedly, hard on the family but some wives get on better if they see their husbands only infrequently.

It is astonishing, looking back on it, what a vast body of work was produced by men who worked in this way and quite often with little or no technical assistance. Leonard Dudgeon at St Thomas's Hospital was not only pathologist to the hospital but carried on a private consulting practice, and in the midst of all these activities managed to do a great deal of fundamental work on immunity. Richard Muir in Glasgow, W. J. Tulloch in Aberdeen, John Eyre at Guys, Ronald Canti at St Bartholomew's, Lionel Whitby at the Middlesex Hospital and many others, all succeeded in doing important research while earning their living in other ways.

Men working in laboratories not connected with hospitals might similarly make their routine duties serve to support their researches. One of them, Dr Fred Griffith, was perhaps the most remarkable of all. His bread and butter was earned by his demarcation of types amongst the streptococci and their application to epidemiological problems in schools and hospitals. This was carried out in the Ministry of Health's laboratory in Endell Sreet off Shaftesbury Avenue, in an ex-workhouse that was even meaner and dirtier than those in the St Mary's Hospital of my student days. Griffith was the titular head of this scientific slum and should therefore have been attending committee meetings and making himself generally useful to the Ministry. Being a shy, retiring bachelor he was utterly incapable of this, for which reason his second in command, Dr W. M. Scott, shouldered these responsibilities. But this enabled Griffith to make, by research whose sheer virtuosity has never been equalled in bacteriology, a discovery whose importance is probably equal to that of penicillin; the part played in genetics by a substance later identified as deoxyribonucleic acid, generally known as D.N.A.

I have gone into this in some detail, not so much to excuse my own shortcomings, but to demonstrate how very recent are the opportunities and facilities now available for anyone wanting to do research. In the days before the war one had to be financially or intellectually abnormal to do it at all.

My own problem was eventually solved, as such things usually are, by something I had not expected: the offer of a post in the Connaught Research Laboratories in Toronto. It meant emigrating. No one called it going down the brain drain in those days. Nor, as is usual at the present time, did I proclaim from the housetops that I was going because the facilities for research were inadequate in this country. I was going for the simple reason that I would soon have no salary, let alone facilities.

As a result, one cold and windy day at the end of August 1936 found us at Liverpool in a tiny cabin, made even smaller by the presence of a large steamer trunk, in the innermost recesses of the *Duchess of Bedford*. Neither of us wanted to go, and our depression was made worse by the fact that most of our fellow passengers were Canadian veterans of the First World War who were even more miserable than we were. They had been present at the unveiling of their memorial on Vimy Ridge and on the outward voyage had been in high spirits with alcohol flowing freely. But by this time they were broke to a man, so broke that they spent most of the voyage in a state of extreme frustration, playing poker for non-existent stakes in front of a bar plentifully supplied with alcohol that none of them could afford.

To add to their misery, and ours, they now remembered what they had temporarily forgotten, that they were going back to a country still in a depression, of whose depth we in England were almost totally unaware. They had no hesitation in telling us what we subsequently found to be only too true, that the prairie provinces which we had always imagined to be roaring with prosperity were literally bankrupt, with a whole year's wheat harvest still unsold and nowhere even to put it.

We celebrated our passage through the Straits of Belle Isle by playing Dvořák's New World Symphony on a portable gramophone in our tiny cabin, and even now the first few bars of the slow movement still bring memories of the desolation of Labrador, the lonely white of the lighthouse and the slow swell of the St Lawrence coming out into the Atlantic. But by the time we had passed Anticosti and saw the cold, clear light of early autumn over the rocks and pines of the Quebec coast, we were beginning to recover our spirits.

They rose still higher when we finally reached Toronto and I first saw my new scientific home. The country might be in a depression and some of it bankrupt, but not the Connaught Laboratories. They were housed in what can only be described as a magnificent building on the campus of the University of Toronto. The entrance was reached by way of double-curving steps, the doors were about 10 feet high, and the entrance hall was constructed largely of marble with Huxley's ideas on a liberal education on one of its walls. The laboratories were equally palatial. One, a magnificent palace, was about 30 feet square but, for all that, inhabited by only one technician. The owner spent most of his time in his office which was larger than the laboratory in which penicillin was discovered.

Still greater men on the staff did not bother with laboratories. They confined their activities to talk and paper work which they conducted in even more luxurious surroundings consisting largely of parquet floors, enormous mahogany desks, carefully selected pictures on the walls and a profusion of potted palms and aspidistras in the corners.

Large and commodious as was the main building, it was only part of the empire. About 10 miles away in the country, there was a large farm with buildings only slightly less elegant than that on the campus. Here it was possible to breed and maintain almost any species of animal. Horses seemed to be the largest but I doubt whether even a hippopotamus would have defeated them – in the summer at least – because there was a suitable stream flowing through the grounds in which it could have wallowed quite happily.

The Connaught Laboratories, given this name for no other reason than that the Duke was Governor-General at the time of its foundation, was nominally part of the University of Toronto. But for all practical purposes it was a separate institution and its own master. It was also very wealthy because, like the Inoculation Department at St Mary's, it made and sold biological products such as insulin, liver extract and vaccines. With the proceeds a great deal of fundamental research was financed. But it was all on a much more prosperous scale, and during the Second World War as many as 900 people were employed at one time.[19]

It also resembled the Inoculation Department in being largely the creation of one man, Dr J. G. Fitzgerald about whom I shall have something to say in the following chapter. He died in 1940, and at the time of the events recorded in this chapter, its Director was Dr R. D. Defries who had been Fitzgerald's assistant from its inception.

I had been asked to go there to study the newly discovered virus of influenza, so that my own activities had little to do with chemotherapy. Nor did I see very much of the new chemotherapy that was developing following the discovery of the sulphonamides, for I had little contact with clinical medicine. The four teaching hospitals in the city were entirely separate institutions, and the only times I went into them were as a visitor or a patient. But I could not help noticing the revolution in medicine that was now starting. Besides puerperal fever, other diseases caused by streptococci such as tonsillitis, scarlet fever, erysipelas, and infections of many wounds had lost their terrors. Diseases caused by other microbes also became amenable to treatment with sulphanilamide. Gonorrhoea, which seldom killed but which could make life extremely uncomfortable, and meningitis, which had previously been almost a sentence of death, could be cut short in a day or so.

If the treatment of bacterial infection was changing rapidly, so was chemotherapy itself. Once the Cinderella of the medical sciences, it had now almost reached the status of Prince Charming. Bacteriologists everywhere almost fell over themselves to pay it court. And so long as it had at least one chemist on its staff, practically every pharmaceutical firm embarked on researches in the hope of discovering new and better sulphonamides – and if possible, ones that could be patented. Chemotherapy had, at last, become not only respectable but big business.

Some of these new sulphonamides could act on microbes unaffected by sulphanilamide. One of the first, sulphapyridine, familiarly known as M and B 693, was synthesized in the cold and winds of the Essex marshes. Perhaps that is why it proved a specific for the treatment of pneumonia. This was followed by a whole series of compounds much too numerous to mention individually that could either deal with other organisms or were less toxic. Nevertheless there remained a great many other species of microbes that were quite unaffected by any of them.

It is not, therefore, surprising that substances bearing no resemblance to the sulphonamides began to be more seriously considered than they had been before their advent. One of them was penicillin. As a result I was brought up with a jolt early in September 1940, when I came across a paper in the *Lancet* dated August 24 by E. Chain, H. W. Florey, A. D. Gardner, N. G. Heatley, M. A. Jennings, A. G. Orr-Ewing, and A. G. Sanders of the Sir William Dunn Laboratory in Oxford with the title, 'Penicillin as a Chemotherapeutic Substance'.[5] It was one of the most astonishing papers I have ever read for it described how they had found a method for its purification, and how to preserve it; they had produced sufficient to demonstrate that it was not only harmless but could protect mice against infection by haemolytic streptococci, staphylococci and one of the species that cause gas gangrene, *Clostridium septicum*.

The method they had used for its purification was not very unlike that employed by Holt. The penicillin in mould juice was extracted with small volumes of amyl acetate after its pH had been dropped to 2·0 with phosphoric acid. The penicillin was then extracted from the amyl acetate solution as the barium salt by mixing it with baryta water at a pH of 6·5–7·0. It was in this way that one of the problems that had defeated previous investigators had been solved.

Further purification and concentration was then carried out involving treatment with charcoal, adsorption in an alumina column, extraction with ether and, finally, production of the sodium salt by careful treatment of the ethereal solution with sodium hydroxide. It was, there is no doubt about it, a masterly piece of work.

The product was then freeze-dried. And it was this that had really saved the day. For, once dried and in a vacuum, it was stable. Without this essential step, the product so laboriously come by would have been as evanescent as its predecessors.

By the time this news reached Toronto the Battle of Britain was reaching its climax, and it seemed more than probable that

Oxford would soon be wiped out, or at best, become German. Under the circumstances the evolution of a compound, that could deal with some of the infections we knew could already be controlled by sulphonamides, seemed an almost unnecessary refinement. Small wonder that I had already forgotten about penicillin by the time the blitz reached London.

What I could not forget was my scientific upbringing. I was, in a sense, a war baby. The whole of my 10 years' apprenticeship with Colebrook, dealing in turn with chemotherapy, puerperal fever and haemolytic streptococci, had been a continuation of the work he had done with Wright and Fleming on infected wounds in France during the First World War. It could even be looked upon as preparation for the war that had now started in earnest. And although I was marooned in Canada studying a virus, my scientific childhood began to assert itself in my thoughts. It had taught me three lessons.

The first was that wounds sustained as a result of enemy action are quite unlike the majority of those produced in the accidents of peacetime, largely because the fragments produced by modern projectiles such as bombs and shells travel at so high a speed that the bones and tissues are smashed to much greater extent than by the objects responsible for most civilian injuries.

The second was that the dead and devitalized tissues exposed in this way form an excellent culture medium for many of the different species of microbes that get into the wound at any time until it is finally healed.

The third was that, with the exception of those organisms responsible for tetanus and gas gangrene, by far the most important were the haemolytic streptococci. Other organisms were much less harmful. They might delay healing and cause scarring but they were not likely to kill the man. The haemolytic streptococci, on the other hand, were much more vicious, producing a rapidly spreading infection with high fever and in many cases septicaemia, which might lead in turn to bronchopneumonia and death. This organism was the outstanding medical problem of the First World War if only because it killed so many men whose wounds were not in themselves serious.

Although such infections were common in all the base

hospitals, they seem to have been at their worst at No 8 Stationary Hospital at Wimereux, where men with compound fractures of the femur were being treated by Major Sinclair. Not, I must hasten to add, because of any fault of his, for he was an expert on this type of injury, but because of the exceptional virulence of the organisms. The state of affairs seems to have been appalling in the summer of 1917. For this reason Fleming with Dr. A. B. Porteous, another member of Wright's team from St Mary's, were sent there and found that over 90 per cent of the wounds were infected by haemolytic streptococci and about half the patients were dying of infection. There was little they could do to treat them but they made attempts to find out how all this had come about. They produced evidence showing that only a minority of the wounds could have acquired these organisms during the journey from the front line but that most of them were due to what we now call cross-infection in the hospital itself. The streptococci were evidently passing from wound to wound.

This work was not published until January 1919 when everyone was trying to forget the horrors of the previous 4 years.[37] To make matters worse the most important piece of information, that dealing with cross-infection, had to wait for the Official History of the War which was not published until long afterwards. Because of all this, very little notice had been taken of all this work.

There was no reason to suppose that the wounds sustained in the war that had now started would be very different from those of the 1914–18 War, that the haemolytic streptococci had lost their virulence in the interval, or that the procedures by which a man was evacuated and treated in hospital were likely to prevent infection any more successfully.

Nevertheless, a great deal had been learned in the meanwhile about the habits of haemolytic streptococci. Could this new knowledge be employed in the present war to prevent some of these infections? The problem could be attacked in two different ways. The organisms might be kept away from the wounds, or they might be destroyed as soon as possible after reaching them.

The first would only be practicable if it could be ascertained where the streptococci had come from and how they travelled to reach the wound. Here, much of the work I had done at Queen Charlotte's came in useful, and shortly before the war started I began to do research, assisted in its later stages by Dr Reba Willits, which resulted in several papers, the first published in the *Lancet* as early as January 1940,[47,50] that confirmed and extended many of Fleming's observations of 22 years before. As a result, it was possible to say with fair confidence that whether the wound had been caused in battle or civil life, it was improbable that the streptococci got into the wound on the object causing it, or on the dust, dirt or pieces of clothing that were driven into it at the time of its infliction, but that they reached it some time later from the nose or throat of anyone who attended it, or from a patient in a neighbouring bed who had an already infected wound.

Although this suggested ways and means of preventing such infections in civil life, there was little hope of their being effective in warfare when large numbers of casualties had to be handled in overcrowded wards with inadequate or unskilled staff.

There remained the second possibility: destruction of the organisms as soon as they reached the wound. Antiseptics had been proved useless for this purpose long before. But in the meanwhile the sulphonamides had made their appearance. Why not fill the wound with sulphanilamide powder and give the man sulphanilamide pills to swallow? This seemed bound to succeed. But most of us had our reservations. Sulphonamides could, for example, be inactivated if the wound contained a great deal of pus. They might possibly be destroyed by some of the other, less dangerous organisms already in the wound. But worst of all, there was the probability that was subsequently proved to be a certainty, that streptococci could become resistant to sulphonamides when used on a large scale.

There was, accordingly, no reason for complacency. History might very well repeat itself when the shooting really started. Such was the state of affairs when, in August 1941, I was suddenly called to the office of Dr R. D. Defries who had become Director of the Connaught Laboratories following the death of Dr Fitzgerald. He introduced me to Prof. Howard Florey and

Dr N. G. Heatley who, he informed me, had been studying a substance called penicillin of which I might possibly have heard.

Florey then told the almost incredible story of how, following the paper to which I have already referred, they had succeeded in producing mould juice in porcelain containers; and how Chain had purified sufficient for the treatment of six moribund patients with staphylococcal infections, only two of whom had died, and even then only because they had run out of penicillin.[1]

It then emerged that the main purpose of their visit was to persuade us to make penicillin in quantity. It was impossible to do so in England. But when we ascertained exactly what this meant, the problem became formidable. Large rooms would be required merely to act as incubators in which to grow the mould. And the method of purification employed at that time seemed difficult to adapt for large-scale production.

The paper describing this work was published on August 16 in the *Lancet*[1] but the journal had not yet reached Toronto for which reason they gave us a typescript copy which I eventually succeeded in purloining. With this in our hands we consulted the chemists. When they asked us how we proposed to produce penicillin, and we told them by growth of the mould in containers of some kind, they laughed at us and predicted that by the time we had spent a great deal of time, money and energy on something so futile, they, the chemists, would have found a way to synthesize it. We must have been unlucky in our choice of chemists because penicillin cannot, even now, be synthesized in any quantity.

We accordingly told Florey that we could not undertake the assignment. He was, naturally, disappointed and I do not think he ever forgave us. But he was, in fact, asking a great deal at that particular stage in the penicillin story. One of the most important requirements was the evolution of a method for large scale production. This was in train already, Florey having found an ally in Dr R. D. Coghill who initiated research for this purpose, and several of the pharmaceutical firms in the United States were diverting men and resources to its study. It seemed unnecessary to duplicate these investigations.[7]

The second requirement was proof of the value of penicillin.

When Florey came to see us, it had only been used for staphylococcal infections. No one knew how it would behave when faced with other organisms under other conditions. I for one had not forgotten how dangerous it is to extrapolate in science, to assume that an agent that will cure infection by one species of microbe will behave in the same way when called upon to deal with other species. The arsenicals had taught me that lesson. But no great quantity of penicillin would be required to set everyone's mind at rest on this matter and it seemed that enough was being made for this purpose.

Such investigations seem to have started in January 1942, by Prof. Florey and Mrs Florey who was also a doctor. They treated 17 severe infections with penicillin administered intravenously and another 172 in which it was applied locally.[41] As more penicillin became available, other workers were called in to help. These included Colebrook, who by this time had reached Glasgow and was investigating burns. Another was J. M. Barnes, also studying burns at Oxford. The Services, too, played their part with Flt. Lt. D. C. Bodenham at Princess Mary's R.A.F. Hospital at Halton, and Col. (now Prof.) R. J. V. Pulvertaft in the Western Desert.

It had been hoped that some at least of the penicillin required for these trials would have come from the United States, but following the holocaust at Pearl Harbour in December 1941, when the American Pacific Fleet was put out of action, even this favour was denied them. It was all kept there and although some was employed for the treatment of casualties in the American army, the fact remains that it was largely with penicillin produced in Britain under appalling conditions of difficulty and frustration that its real value in the treatment of war wounds was proved.

As a result of all this it gradually became clear that, as we had suspected from the beginning, the sulphonamides had such limitations that they were very nearly useless. Although of undoubted value in diseases such as pneumonia where only one microbe was involved, the conditions they had to face in a large open wound infected by a variety of different organisms in the presence of pus and dead or devitalized tissues were far beyond their capabilities. Had the invasion of Europe occurred in 1942, there seems little doubt that some of the base hospitals would have been similar to those in the First World War, with long rows of men desperately ill with severe and uncontrollable infections of their wounds.

The investigations carried out so carefully in 1942 showed clearly that penicillin possessed properties denied to the sulphonamides. Provided large enough doses could be given, it could deal with heavily infected wounds. But, far more important, if applied locally soon after the wound had been inflicted, it could prevent infection of any severity developing at all. This was amply demonstrated during a visit Florey paid to Africa in 1943, when it was found that, provided penicillin could be instilled into the wound, it could actually be closed soon after infliction. So different was this from all previous practice that few surgeons believed it was possible – until they saw the results.[39]

If, as seemed probable, this would become standard practice in the battles to come, enormous quantities of penicillin would be required. We all knew that, given time, means would be found for producing the large volumes of mould juice required as raw material by deep fermentation in large tanks. But although attempts were being made to do this on both sides of the Atlantic, rumour had it that formidable difficulties were being encountered. The wounded could not wait for them to be overcome. The only alternative was the method Ridley and Craddock had used in 1929; growth of the mould in shallow layers of broth in containers of some kind, expensive and time-consuming though it might be.

Since the Connaught Laboratories, with their experience of macro-methods behind them, would undoubtedly have to play a part in exercises of this nature, it was from that time onwards tacitly assumed that, for no other reason than that I had been engaged in extra-mural researches on wound infections when my real function about the place was study of the virus of influenza, and the even more specious reason that I had witnessed the discovery of penicillin, I would be the Pooh Bah to make it when the time came. In the meanwhile Dr Philip Greey, who was a member of the Department of Bacteriology in the University, began to produce as much mould juice as his facilities permitted. It was given to Dr F. S. Macdonald, a young chemist on the staff of Prof. Charles H. Best in the Banting Institute, who evolved a method of extraction based on that used by Chain. In this way they learned a great deal about the vagaries of penicillin production and, because that which they produced was used for the treatment of patients in the Toronto General Hospital, something about its value.

It was because of this fate in store for me that I was sent with Greey, early in 1943, to visit the Northern Agricultural Research Laboratory at Peoria in Illinois, about 100 miles west of Chicago. Here were collected the brains of penicillin production in the United States. It was probably because of this that the building was so well protected against intruders for we found its entrance guarded by a uniformed individual looking rather like a cowboy, attached to an enormous holster from which a six-shooter protruded. But after we had given our names, had large labels pinned on our lapels proclaiming who we were, and the presiding deity had signified over the telephone his willingness to receive us, the cowboy had no compunction about leaving the entrance completely unguarded while he conducted us to our hosts.

Perhaps the most important outcome of our visit was the information given us by Dr A. J. Moyer that corn steep liquor was an elixir which, when added to the medium, increased the production of penicillin to almost astronomical heights. Neither of us had ever heard of it before, but it appeared that it was a by-product of any manufacturing process that employed corn as a raw material. Before anything could be done with it, the hard outer coating had first to be removed by treatment with sodium sulphite. The resulting liquor containing this coat, with the starch adhering to it, yields after evaporation a dark brown liquid with a marked taste of toffee. Large quantities were apparently available, mostly because no one knew what to do with it. Dr Moyer kindly gave us a medicine bottle full of it but warned us that the cowboy was a simple-minded soul who had been warned that nothing was to be taken from the building. He advised us to hide it. And so, clutching our little bottle in the pocket of one of our mackintoshes, we went down to the entrance. It was, once again, unguarded. The cowboy had gone, this time to lunch, taking his six-shooter with him.

Shortly before this, Chain's laboratory in Oxford had begun to process mould juice sent in milk churns from Kemball Bishop and Co., whose factory at Bromley by Bow had survived the bombing. Several other commercial firms soon took part in these activities, which are admirably described in a little book by Mr David Masters.[60] As a result, comparatively large amounts of penicillin were ultimately made in Great Britain.

Somewhat similar arrangements, but on a much larger scale, were made in the United States so that during 1943 no less than twenty factories began to produce penicillin. Many were installed in the premises of the larger manufacturing chemists but some were comparatively small. One was so successful an adaptation of a plant for the production of mushroom spawn that, for a time, its owner was looked upon as the coming man in the industry. But some were started by amateurs who seemed to be doing it as much for fun as from patriotic or pecuniary motives. One was in a shop in the main street of a little country town with a basement full of inflammable liquids, and was the worst fire trap I have ever seen. Perhaps that is why the chemist in charge of it chewed gum the whole of the three hours we were with him. But the most remarkable was run by a business-man employing a bacteriological technique entirely his own invention, based mostly on old whisky bottles sterilized by steam direct from a boiler on the point of bursting, in the Stygian gloom of a derelict factory in the meaner part of Brooklyn, and staffed entirely by negresses. Unorthodox some of them may have been, but the fact remains that the Americans got their penicillin.

Canadian needs were met by a pharmaceutical firm in Montreal and the Connaught Laboratories. Its Director at the time, Dr R. D. Defries has written a full description of how the latter coped with the problem.[19] What follows is a more personal account of the activities of the three amateurs directly concerned, Greey, Macdonald and myself who, despite the fact that we had the haziest notion how to do it, were told to make penicillin to the tune of 50,000,000 units a day, and to have some ready for D-Day which we all knew would be some time next summer.

One of the first requirements was space. No less than 8,000 square feet would be required for the incubator rooms alone. The Connaught itself could not possibly provide so much. Several repulsive-looking factories were inspected, but in the end something almost on the doorstep was found which, although far from ideal, did at least provide enough room. So much, that half the building was straightaway appropriated for another major Connaught activity at that time, the freeze drying of human serum for the treatment of shock.

The building we had acquired in this way was generally known as Old Knox College. It had originally been built as a seminary for the training of Presbyterian clergymen. But when the amalgamation of a number of different colleges was achieved to make the University of Toronto the educational establishment it is now, a new Knox College was built on the campus. The old building then began a somewhat chequered career but which generally had something medical about it. It accordingly did duty as a military hospital during the First World War and then became the headquarters of the Health Department of Ontario. But when the latter moved to a large building in Queen's Park it was left uninhabited for many years.

Having been originally built in 1874 it was, for Toronto, almost an ancient monument. It had a high central tower, steep roofs broken by chimneys, and dormer windows all embellished with large quantities of ornamental iron. It had a profusion of long narrow windows under stone arches and quite an imposing entrance approached by stone steps. Situated in the centre of an open space and some distance from the nearest buildings, it faced south down the wide expanse of Spadina Avenue towards the lake. Altogether it possessed a great deal of charm and dignity.

It was as firm as a rock, having been built of brick at a time when buildings were meant to last. But it had become extremely dilapidated and would require a great deal of renovation both inside and out. This did not matter and its owner was delighted to get it off his hands. And so, in September 1943, we acquired somewhere to make penicillin. Architects were installed in rooms at the back of the building whose floors seemed to be the only safe specimens in the building. Even so they were less safe than they appeared to be, for several weeks after the architects had taken up residence some tubes of nitro-glycerine, a legacy from a previous tenant, were found in the rooms below. The enormous Scottish foreman who discovered them was trembling so much that I thought he might drop them. Fortunately, a bucket of water was handy and the police eventually sank them in the lake.

The building did, it is true, provide the space required. But that is about the best that could be said for it. Except for the fact that the chemical extraction plant could, with considerable difficulty, be squeezed into some vaults that had, at one time, housed the vital statistics of Ontario, and that the sterilizers were easily accommodated in a large room on the first floor that had probably done duty as a public health laboratory, the rest of the factory was dispersed over three floors, and in rooms none of which were ideal for the purpose. Some of the floors had to be strengthened by steel posts and girders. And an enormous lift had to be installed to carry the containers in which the mould juice was produced. Most of the rooms were converted into incubators in which to grow the mould. Their internal temperature was a matter of very considerable importance. It had to be kept exactly at 75·5°F (24°C) so that the windows had to be blacked out to exclude the sun which, in the summer, would have made their temperature much too high. Even so, an enormous air-conditioning plant had to be installed in the basement with yards of air ducts going to each of the rooms. The basement itself was a new construction. It had to be excavated and the footings of the walls deepened to provide the necessary head-room. Altogether, it was an operation of considerable magnitude.

Procuring the apparatus we required was also a complicated operation. Everything was in short supply and many essentials were governed by priorities. Moreover, most of it had to come from the United States. To facilitate all this, all the Canadian and American factories were not only given top priority but placed under the orders of a Dictator of Penicillin in Washington. He had to approve of everything we did or required. We were, for a time, mortally afraid of him.

Early in the proceedings we went to Washington to make his

acquaintance. Taking with us most of the administration of the laboratories we hired a room at an hotel, deposited them in it, and a small deputation repaired to the lobby to await his arrival. As befits a Dictator he was late, and as the minutes passed we gradually became more and more speechless with apprehension. After what seemed aeons of time there was a scream of brakes at the door, and a little man rushed in. He was sorry he was late but explained that his penicillin commitments had kept him up until 4.00 a.m. Fortunately, he had nothing to complain about and in due time we repaired for lunch. Asked what he would have, he never even bothered to look at the menu but demanded a martini and baked ham.

The baked ham was simple but the martini posed a problem. Although prohibition in Canada had been revoked 10 years before, the consumption of alcohol on the premises of the University of Toronto was still forbidden. In consequence, student dances at Hart House, the University recreational centre, were officially devoid of alcohol. Unofficially they were anything but that, for the dancers spent a considerable amount of their time in the cars parked outside, consuming enough refreshment to enable them to enjoy the party.

Another consequence of this embargo was that official pilgrimages by representatives of the Connaught, which prided itself on being part of the University despite its commercial activities, were seldom lubricated by alcohol. There was, accordingly, danger that the Dictator might have to consume his martini alone while the rest of us made do with iced water. But the fact that the future of penicillin obviously depended on one man's whim, the fact that we were on neutral territory and that I felt the need of alcoholic refreshment as much as the Dictator, prompted me to order a baked ham and martini as well. Despite glares of disapproval from the more hidebound, some of the rest followed suit and we had quite a jolly party. I wonder how many Canadian soldiers owe their lives to the mollifying influence of gin in Washington.

Now that we had a home we could get down to business. Our main preoccupation was time. It was already October, so that there was no time for experimentation. We had to go straight from the drawing board to horribly permanent bricks and mortar and woe betide us if we forgot something, or it failed to work, or did not fit.

One of our first problems was the type of container in which the mould was to be grown. There were two schools of thought. One favoured large trays, and the other bottles or flasks. At the beginning we were all for trays, but towards the end of November Macdonald arrived back from Washington with the news that trays had been found to be unsatisfactory. It would be better if we changed to bottles. This was serious because the equipment, the autoclaves and even the layout of the building would all have to be altered. Then began about a fortnight of the most feverish activity I have ever encountered.

The worst problem was the building. Having been originally designed for the training of Presbyterian clergymen, to whom a few steps here and there did not matter, we had had to tinker with the floor levels in order to ensure smooth passage of the trays. Bottles, however, would require a different set of levels. And the concrete mixer was already in position and about to pour some of the floors. Fortunately, the clerk of the works was a Gaelic-speaking Highlander, who apparently entertained his daughter every evening by giving her mathematical problems to solve but was not devoid of a sense of humour. He persuaded the man who operated the concrete mixer to take a day or two off while we were closeted with the architects. They, too, were co-operative, if only because their chief draughtsman was at heart an artist and he only drew plans to enable him to eat; the more he drew the better nourished he was.

The bottles we used were about the same overall dimensions as a milk-bottle, but with longer sides and more rounded shoulders. We required 250,000 of them. So many, that until we started to use them, the only place big enough to store them was under the stands in the University football ground. When in use, they were incubated lying on their sides to provide a shallow layer of broth. As they contained only 150 c.c. (5 ounces) of medium, we had to deal with about 30,000 of them every 24 hours. They each weighed about $1\frac{1}{2}$ lb., so that the total weight was about 20 tons.

If this were not enough, each bottle went through no less than twelve different processes. At the end of incubation they had to be taken off the incubator racks, put on to transport racks, wheeled to the emptying tank (which sometimes involved a journey by lift) where they were emptied, washed, filled with new medium, plugged with wool, sterilized, cooled, inoculated with spores, transported to the incubator rooms and piled once more on the racks.

All this meant that each bottle was actually handled by human hands no less than five different times. But we were able to mechanize some stages by using dairy equipment such as a washing machine, a filling machine, and moving belts for their transportation. But most of their journeys were on metal racks we had to design ourselves. And the trolleys on which the latter were carried were, we considered, one of our masterpieces.

Extraction of the penicillin from the mould juice, which had been such a problem for the pioneers, was no longer a difficulty. It had become more or less standardized. Its most important step was simple – mixture of ice-cold mould juice with phosphoric acid and amyl acetate in such a way that, within a few seconds, it ran into a large centrifuge similar to those used for the separation of cream from milk. As a result, penicillin went into solution in the amyl acetate and came out of the spout labelled 'cream' while the acid broth denuded of its penicillin went out of the other spout labelled 'milk' and down the drain.

The extraction of the penicillin from the amyl acetate was effected by mixing it with weak alkali. There were, of course, further steps before it was fit for use. These were no problem and the resulting product was freeze dried.

Since we would be harvesting nearly 1,000 gallons of mould juice every day, the apparatus had to be on a very different scale from the 4-litre flask perched precariously on a draining board that had sufficed for Ridley and Craddock. A great many tanks would be needed, all made of stainless steel – penicillin, it seemed, was still unstable enough to object to baser metals – not to mention what seemed like several miles of piping made from the same material. Four enormous milk separators, a great many electric motors and pumps, and no less than 20 tons of refrigeration, whose machine must have weighed all of that, would also be necessary.

The fitting together of all this complicated mass of machinery was left to Macdonald and his assistant, Dr N. L. Macpherson, a broad-shouldered Scotsman who was a chemical engineer by profession. So far as I could see, most of their planning was done on the back of old envelopes. But done it was, on time, and with little to alter when they started to use it.

Shortly after Christmas the Dictator of Penicillin signified his intention of calling upon us. He was to arrive in an aeroplane provided by the American forces. We accordingly met him at Malton airport, at that time no more than a hut on the edge of a large field. He was accompanied by a large bundle which, he explained, was a parachute. Surprised that key officials were apparently transported in aeroplanes of doubtful stability, we counted ourselves fortunate in having brought the largest and safest of the cars available. Even so, parachutes are valueless as life-savers on a modern motorway, for which reason the driver refrained from excessive speed on the way into Toronto; so much so, that the Dictator was beginning to exhibit signs of impatience as we wended our leisurely way along the lakeside. But fortunately we soon turned north; and, mounting the steep incline of the bridge over the railway tracks, came to the summit. There before us, half a mile away at the end of the wide vista provided by Spadina Avenue – at this distance looking almost prosperous – there were the towers and turrets, the steep roofs and the many-windowed wings of Old Knox College, the home of Torontian penicillin. Even Dictators retain sufficient humility to be impressed.

At dinner that evening, the licensing laws of Ontario prevented our offering him a martini. He had to make do with an indifferent sherry. He also had to make do with a less luxurious mode of transport than an aeroplane when he left later in the evening for Montreal. That which had brought him was, I suppose, not only lacking in stability but ability to find its way by night, for he took the train like everyone else. But unlike them, with a large parachute for bedfellow.

As the building of the plant and the installation of the

machinery progressed, we had to start thinking about its operation. From the start, it had been planned for it to operate 24 hours a day for 7 days a week. The recruitment and training of the nearly 100 workers prepared to do it was by no means easy. Since it was now 1944 we could not afford to pick and choose, so that we acquired some very doubtful characters. There was a suspicion that one had been in prison, another who was a diabetic chose to go into coma on a catwalk high up over moving machinery, and a third, obviously a schizophrenic, began to exhibit homicidal tendencies.

Essential supplies were not always easy to obtain. We only succeeded in getting sufficient bottles by accident. The manufacturers in Chicago had told their sales department to refuse further orders. Fortunately, ours were ordered by telephone while the man in charge was out at lunch. His deputy, being unaware of the change in policy and no doubt pleased at the prospect of promotion that would come as a result of his salesmanship in taking an order for a quarter of a million bottles, duly accepted the order. He was more probably sacked; but, with a stern warning that these were all we would get, they accepted the order. Corn steep liquor, too, we had been told, was in abundance and difficult to get rid of because no one wanted it. But it seemed very difficult to extract from the factory in Quebec, and on one occasion we were down to one barrel. Lactose, whose only source is milk, could only be obtained in sufficient quantity when the Controller of Boilers in Ottawa was prevailed upon to allow a cheese manufacturer to have a larger one so that he could step up his production of cheese and so provide himself with sufficient whey from which to extract the lactose we required.

Even when everything was in place, the staff hired and trained, and adequate supplies forthcoming, we still had our problems. When we started we naturally employed only one shift in every 24 hours. But when we began to step up production by starting another, and shortly afterwards a third, production did not treble. It remained more or less the same as with only one shift. We held several meetings to find out why. The bacteriologists accused the chemists of losing penicillin in the extraction process. The chemists retaliated by suggesting that the bacteriologists were not producing it. The proceedings became acrimonious until someone produced a compromise; that the penicillin was inactivated while flowing down about 6 feet of pipe from the bacteriologists to the chemists. So obsessed were we by the instability of penicillin that we almost welcomed this explanation. It took us a long time to find the real reason: that the more bottles we piled into the incubator rooms, the more likely they were to overheat and destroy the penicillin as soon as it was formed. All we had to do was to install large fans to get the air moving, and the production of penicillin rose accordingly.

This is the barest outline of how three amateurs, helped enormously by Dr R. D. Defries, the Director of the Laboratories, and Col. A. D. LePan, the Building Superintendent of the University, succeeded in building a factory, staffing it and getting production going. And on April 26, 1944, the first penicillin came off the production line – 20,000,000 units in about a litre of fluid. Unfortunately it smelt strongly of goats, due to traces of caprylic alcohol the chemists had used to prevent frothing. It had to be re-processed. Succeeding batches were less goaty but, even so, bore little resemblance to the pure white substance that is nowadays injected into our anatomy. But they did contain penicillin, and on May 20 our first vials containing the dirty-yellow powder were accepted by the Government of Canada.

We had done it, but only just. Canadian troops landed in Normandy on D-Day, June 6, exactly 17 days later, with, I hope, Canadian penicillin in their medical equipment.

Penicillin proved itself in the subsequent battles on the Continent. It stopped the almost inevitable sepsis that would have been the lot of so many of the wounded who had been saved from death by the newly introduced methods for dealing with shock and haemorrhage. The number of men who owe their lives to it has never been counted but it must be many thousands.

There can be very little doubt that, but for Florey, none of this would have come about. It was entirely as a result of his initiative that penicillin was found to be of value in the first place. It was his persistence that induced others to make it in quantity and his advocacy of early treatment with it, and closure of the wounds soon after infliction, that prevented a repetition of the dreadful conditions of the wounded at No. 8 Stationary Hospital at Wimereux in the First World War.

In all this, Fleming played virtually no part at all. But by a strange whim of fate it was he who captured the imagination of the public to an almost unbelievable extent. And what is more, it happened almost overnight, following the publication of an editorial by *The Times* on August 27, 1942. The reason for this incursion into chemotherapy on the part of a daily newspaper was that Fleming had treated and cured a patient in St Mary's Hospital who was dying of streptococcal meningitis, with penicillin given him by Florey and which was all he possessed at that time. The editorial referred to this case as an example of what a new compound, of which the public had hitherto been quite unaware, could do. But it omitted to mention either Fleming or Florey. Wright thereupon wrote a letter to *The Times* drawing attention to the fact that penicillin had been discovered by Fleming. He omitted to mention Florey but included – he could never resist the temptation – a Latin tag, *palmam qui meruit ferat*.

The storm broke. Almost overnight, Fleming became famous. He was undoubtedly helped by the fact that few exercises commend themselves more to the British public than discrediting the medical profession. They had done it again. They had had in their midst an inarticulate Scot who had discovered a new substance worth its weight in gold but which none of them would have anything to do with for 12 long years. Once again they had been caught napping. They had failed to recognize a good thing when they saw it.

Small wonder, therefore, that when Fleming came to America in the summer of 1945 he made what can only be described as a triumphal progress. Some time before his arrival he had already been given one of the highest honours the Americans could give him, his portrait in colour on the cover of *Time* magazine; but when he got there he received another, several pages of the *New Yorker* devoted to an account of an interview with one of its reporters. But the real accolade was given him when he reached Boston and was awarded an honorary degree by Harvard University. The other recipient was General Marshall. It was not the soldier but the little Scot who received the bigger ovation.

Despite this, he came to Toronto to see us. He arrived one sweltering day in July arrayed in the thickest pair of flannel trousers I have ever seen, and a jacket made of Harris tweed more suitable for wear in its homeland than in Toronto in summer. But he was as cool as a cucumber. His main purpose in coming to Toronto, so he informed me soon after his arrival, was to buy a pair of English shoes. Shoes made in England were, apparently, not to be had there, even by the discoverer of penicillin.

His fame had not spoiled him. He was the same silent, dour Scot he had always been. We dined him and wined him to the best of our ability, and we took him to inspect the penicillin factory. As I had expected, he never even hinted that it was a creditable achievement. It was no more than what was to be expected of an old boy of the Inoculation Department.

And so, in company with Mr John Cameron of the Ministry of Supply who was acting as his amanuensis, we took him down to the station in the derelict Ford V8 we had bought second-hand 6 years previously, and put him on the train for Montreal. Not long afterwards he went to Stockholm to receive the Nobel Prize.

Chapter 10

An Ounce of Prevention

Like that of all medical men, my training as a student had been directed towards making me sufficiently competent to diagnose and treat human disease. After I qualified, my activities were very much the same even though they concerned only one disease. But although a high proportion of the profession practise medicine in this way and with the same objectives, this is not the whole of medicine. Quite a number of diseases can be prevented from occurring at all. Scurvy, for example, can be prevented by an adequate diet, malaria by control of mosquitoes, and goitre by adding iodine to the table salt. Equally successful are methods that were introduced when the connection between microbes and human disease was finally established. This was largely because the prevention of such diseases is frequently possible if the lines of communication along which the microbes travel from their sources to their victims can be cut or, alternatively, potential victims rendered so resistant to infection that the microbes, even if they get to them, are unable to do them harm.

Important as this may be, the general practitioner and the medical, surgical or obstetric specialist can play only a small part in the prevention of infection by such methods, for they frequently require techniques that are very different from those employed for curing disease. They include the planning and building of major engineering projects such as sewage disposal systems, reservoirs and the draining of marshes. They may also entail the supervision of inspectors to control the purity of food and milk, health visitors who keep an eye on the well-being of children in the community, and immunization for the prevention of infectious disease. To do all this requires the training and employment of large numbers of medical men whose activities constitute a discipline that is very different from curative medicine.

This form of medicine has never acquired a very satisfactory nomenclature. Over the years, it has been called Public Health, Hygiene, Social Medicine and, more recently, Community Medicine. But by far the best, if only because it describes its ultimate objective, is Preventive Medicine. For this reason alone, not to mention the different techniques employed, those who practise it are almost automatically cut off from the main body of medical thought and procedures.

Some of the medical sciences have, however, a foot in both camps: bacteriology in particular, because microbial diseases not only lend themselves more readily than most to prevention but also because many of them can, nowadays, be cured. Even so, few bacteriologists can be equally skilled in the bacteriology of both curative and preventive medicine. And although the hospital bacteriologist has much to do with the diagnosis of bacterial infection and its treatment, any attempts he may make towards its prevention may amount to no more than control of cross-infection in wards and the supervision of the sterilizing procedures in his hospital. On the other hand the public health bacteriologist may know a great deal about the microbes in water, sewage and milk, their behaviour in large populations and the immunization of such populations by vaccines, but next to nothing about the treatment of patients with antibiotics or the sterilization of dressings.

Until I arrived in Canada I had always considered myself to be an inhabitant of the curative camp, and that since I had been hired by the Connaught Laboratories which had a considerable reputation for fundamental research and made products such as insulin and liver extract with which to treat disease, I had every reason for supposing that I would remain in the same camp. But, within a few minutes of entering my new home for the first time, I was handed a note saying that I had been appointed a Lecturer in the Department of Hygiene and Preventive Medicine in the Faculty of Medicine and that my emolument would be 200 dollars per annum. Although grateful for the increase in salary within so short a space of time, I little realized the full impact this brief note would have on my activities, and that it would involve my becoming a permanent inhabitant of the opposite camp for the next 10 years. How this came about, and what I did, form the subject of this chapter.

I did not have long to wait before I gained some inkling of the fate in store for me, because within an hour of my receiving the fateful note it was intimated that I should attend the Field Course. Not having the slightest idea of what constituted a Field Course, but unwilling to reveal my ignorance of what appeared to be common knowledge in Toronto, it was some time before I discovered that the Field Course was a ceremony compulsorily attended by the fifth-year medical students. It started within a week of my arrival and turned out to be a course of instruction on the practical aspects of public health. The students were shown how to prevent disease by the appropriate methods, so that when they went into practice in the more remote parts of the Dominion they could act as part-time, very amateur public health officers in addition to their normal duties as general practitioners. Instruction of this type was excellent but, unfortunately, the 3 weeks required for it should have been the last 3 weeks of their holidays. This might not have excited comment in England, where holidays during the clinical years of the medical course have to be snatched whenever time becomes available. But it was a serious matter to a Canadian student, because most of them depended on what they could earn during the long vacation that lasted from May until the beginning of October, in order to pay for their board and lodging during the following winter. The loss of 3 weeks wages was no light matter. This was bad enough, but far from the students being interested in the practice of preventive medicine, they were violently opposed to the whole business. They all had a vested interest in disease. Within a year or so it would be their sole source of income, so that the less that was prevented the better.

As a result, long before I had found my way about, I spent most of my days in company with 120 sullen, unwilling students being lectured on such improving subjects as the most efficient methods for the disposal of the human metabolism, the exact number of lumens that are required to enable one to read by artificial light, and the virtues of immunization against such diseases as yellow fever which never occur in Canada.

Most of our instruction consisted of visits to such salubrious places as sewage farms, the archives where the Province of Ontario kept track of its inhabitants, the incinerator in which the garbage of Toronto was disposed of, and the plant on the island which abstracts water from Lake Ontario by a pipe, which had inadvertently been placed so close to the sewage outfall that the purification system must have been of quite remarkable efficiency. Schools catering for both normal children and those suffering from various forms of defect were also on the itinerary, as were factories whose procedures lent themselves to mutilation of the operatives. By way of light relief we accompanied sanitary inspectors on their rounds to see to what depths of depravity Canadian landlords might have descended, and to restaurants to plunge thermometers into the washing-up water to determine whether it was hot enough. We also inspected milk pasteurizing and bottling factories and, leaving nothing to the imagination, the dairy farms that produced the raw material. One was so advanced that the cows were milked to music and the hens were dyed pink for a reason that escapes me. But we were brought back to reality by a visit to an abattoir where bullocks enter at one end and emerge as sausages at the other. Strange as it may seem, no student ever got mixed up in the assembly line to such an extent that he emerged as a sausage, but we had some narrow escapes.

All this was bad enough, but every student had been given a loose-leaf book containing mimeographed sheets with large spaces, which he was expected to fill in during his evening leisure hours. In this way it was hoped that the instruction imparted during the day would not only become fixed in his memory, but he would treasure the book for the rest of his life and refer to it in crises of a public health nature in his practice. Unfortunately, many of the questions could only be answered by someone with a lifetime of experience of public health in general, and that of Ontario in particular. And even when they were expected to describe a process they had actually seen, they were seriously handicapped by the simple fact that the environment had invariably been very noisy, and the demonstrator a very small man with a very small voice who had confined his remarks to the dozen or so students in his immediate vicinity.

These books were supposed to be filled in and delivered to the authorities at the end of the course, and eventually a batch of about twenty appeared on my desk. I was expected to read each of their hundred or more pages, correct mistakes and allot marks. Not knowing anything whatever about the public health procedures of my new homeland, I picked out the one or two items about which I had a smattering and read them. I read the same items in a second book, and again in a third. By this time I had become aware that the language seemed strangely familiar. No wonder, for it was identical in all three.

Puzzled by this extraordinary unanimity, I enquired the reason of one of my colleagues. The explanation was simple. Practically every fraternity house, in which most of the students lived, had acquired one of these books which some long-forgotten alumnus had succeeded in filling in. All that the present generation had to do was to copy the information into theirs. Whether it was correct and up to date did not seem to matter. The practice had, at least, one merit. One need not read any of the books. One merely gave all of them enough marks to pass. Even so, the pile of books invariably cluttered one's desk for months before one could bring oneself to do even as much as this.

Thus, within a month of my arrival in Canada, ostensibly to further the art and science of bacteriology, I became aware that I had spent practically all my time learning an entirely new subject a great deal of which seemed to have little to do with bacteriology. I was at first puzzled by this, but consoled myself by the fact that I was being paid 200 dollars a year for doing so. What I had not realized was that the man who had hired me, Dr J. G. Fitzgerald, was not only Director of the Connaught Laboratories but also Professor of Hygiene and Preventive Medicine in the University and that it was because I was a member of his staff that I was participating in such non-bacteriological activities. And it was not long before I became aware that

I would soon have to learn considerably more about the subject because Fitzgerald had become dissatisfied with the method of teaching in his department.

He had come to the conclusion that the old system of didactic lectures – a term much used in Toronto – was useless. It entailed the 120 students sitting for an hour, asleep, doodling, reading or merely vegetating while some unhappy lecturer strained every nerve to interest them in a subject for which they had no regard whatever. Henceforth, they were to be intensively instructed. So intensively that they were, so to speak, to instruct themselves by giving short lecturettes on some aspect of preventive medicine which would then be debated by the class and lecturer. Spare-time study and especially the reading of books and scientific communications was also required. To achieve all this, the class was split into groups of about twenty students each of which was delivered, lock, stock and barrel, to the tender mercies of one lecturer twice a week for about 4 months.

The other five instructors were, of course, well acquainted with the subject. Two of them were full professors and the remainder were well up the academic ladder. I was nowhere in this galaxy of talent. All that I knew about the subject were the remnants of what I had picked up as long before as 1921 while attending a series of lectures that were unlike any of the others given to us as students. In the first place, attendance was compulsory; the examining bodies required it, not because of their unusual regard for preventive medicine, but because the particular professional body to which its devotees belonged objected to its members suffering the indignity of lecturing to empty benches. In the second place, the lectures were delivered at 9.00 a.m. on Saturdays in the summer term. Further comment on this is unnecessary. But even so, compulsory attendance and the unfortunate timing of the lectures might have been condoned had they been worth attending. They were not. For the choice of lecturer to give them was also unfortunate. He was not only inarticulate, but so shy that he could not even look at his audience. Nor was the subject inspiring for it seemed to concern drains, the disposal of garbage and the notification of infectious diseases, interspersed with statistics that may have been vital but which the lecturer succeeded in making completely lifeless.

With this as my only training for a course of about thirty lectures, it became necessary for me to spend a considerable amount of my time trying to keep at least one lecture ahead of my class. Even so, the difficulties were formidable because there were neither syllabus nor text book to provide guidance. Nor was I assisted in any way by my pupils. For although the theory on which their education was founded may have been excellent, they never did what the theory expected of them. No student, so far as I could make out, ever did any spare-time reading whatever, and even when told to prepare a lecturette was either absent when he should have delivered it or pleaded pressure of other duties. Even simple question and answer was useless because none of them knew anything whatever about the subject.

In the end I think most of us gave up the struggle and imparted the instruction in the same way as before the experiment started, in a series of didactic lectures. But instead of only one lecturer wasting his time, six of us did so simultaneously.

For a time, some of us were optimistic enough to hope that we would soon be rid of this incubus because its originator was dispatched by the Rockefeller Foundation to make an extended tour of Europe, that took him as far afield as Moscow, in order to report on the methods of teaching preventive medicine employed in the Old World. He returned in due course and reported what we hoped he would not: that praiseworthy as the efforts of the European instructors might be, the teaching of preventive medicine was nowhere up to the standard of Toronto where the method of teaching could not be bettered.

In view of this mass of evidence our chief had collected in support of his theories of education, it is perhaps not surprising that none of us dare express our feelings on the subject. But he died in 1940, the war began in earnest about the same time, and it was suddenly discovered that the intensive teaching of preventive medicine to medical students could, perhaps, be postponed until more peaceful conditions returned. The scheme was quietly dropped, without, so far as I know any serious deterioration in the health of the Dominion.

It should be obvious that a man who succeeded in robbing the students of 3 weeks vacation, and compelling six or seven members of his staff to spend so much of their time with so little to show for it, was no ordinary person. Dr J. G. Fitzgerald was quite as remarkable a man as any of those I have mentioned in the preceding pages. Qualifying in 1903 at the University of Toronto, he had for a time dabbled in psychiatry but soon became interested in bacteriology. He worked in several Continental laboratories including the Pasteur Institutes of Paris and Brussels under such great men as Roux and Bordet. He then returned to Toronto in 1913.

By this time he had learned two lessons that were to mould his actions for the rest of his life. The first was that a great many diseases could already be prevented, that some could be cured, and that both would soon be possible in many other diseases. The second was that to do so costs money that all too often the individual household cannot afford, largely because the remedies required may not only be intrinsically expensive but made more so by their having to be produced by profit-making commercial houses. He accordingly set out to do what he could to right the situation.

Partly because he was himself a bacteriologist and partly because diphtheria antitoxin could cure the disease, he began by producing it in five horses stabled in a galvanized iron shed on the outskirts of Toronto. The serum was concentrated and purified in the basement of the medical school in the city. In this way, he was able to produce a known remedy for a disease at a price far below that charged by commercial houses. With this inducement, Provincial Boards of Health (health in Canada is largely a Provincial and not a Federal responsibility) were persuaded to buy it and issue it free of charge for the treatment of cases of the disease wherever they might occur.

This may seem very ordinary nowadays, but we must remember that this was before the First World War when disease meant that someone had to pay the doctor for treating it. It was therefore a revolutionary procedure in Canada. But it had immense consequences.

One was the metamorphosis of the small organization Fitzgerald had created in this way, into the Connaught Laboratories, part of, but virtually independent of, the University of Toronto. For a time it was housed in a comparatively small building at the farm on the outskirts of Toronto, but before very long most of its activities were transferred to the large building on the campus of the University, which it shared with the School of Hygiene.

As a result of the precedent he had established in the case of diphtheria antitoxin, he undertook the manufacture of a whole series of agents for free distribution to doctors by Provincial Boards of Health all over Canada, so that by the time I arrived on the scene they included insulin, liver extract, adrenalin and a great many bacteriological products. The money obtained in this way was ploughed back into research and teaching in the Connaught and the School of Hygiene. Contrary to what might have been expected, very little of this research had to do with the products intended for the treatment of established disease. Fitzgerald was much more interested in research that would lead to its prevention and to facilitate this had been appointed Professor of Hygiene and Preventive Medicine in the University soon after the First World War. As he remained Director of the Connaught Laboratories, there was no difficulty about making funds available for the prevention rather than the cure of disease.

It was because of this that, without my realizing it, I was translated from the camp of curative bacteriologists to that inhabited by the preventives almost as soon as I arrived. What is more, by great good fortune, I found myself in one of the principal centres of teaching and research on preventive medicine. Like the Inoculation Department that knew more about the treatment of microbial disease, I was now in an institution that knew more than anyone else about its prevention.

It is therefore praiseworthy that this practice began, so to speak, at home, presumably to set an example to the rest of the University and the country at large.

All of us were, for example, subjected to an annual medical examination in order to detect and if possible correct any serious deviations from the normal in our natural functions so that they could be corrected before they became permanent and irreversible. Although good in theory, it left much to be desired in practice; so much so that the only serious illnesses that occurred were, as it happened, of such a character that they could not have been detected no matter how skilled the examiners, or alternatively there was no way of treating them. When, therefore, the individual responsible for the examinations went to the war, it was suddenly discovered that we all had better things to do and the scheme was dropped.

Other more domestic measures were also employed to keep us healthy. They mostly concerned minute attention to diet and insistence on the importance of recreation.

Diet was largely attended to by the serving of a nutritious and carefully balanced lunch every day, which had been compounded by a fully trained dietician. Suitable accommodation was accordingly provided in a very pleasant room on the top floor. The lunch consisted of soup, entrée, sweet, and coffee or milk. It was actually a very good lunch and cheap at the price. But the absence of any luckless wight who preferred sandwiches in the park, a glass of beer at a pub or wanted to lunch at home with his wife, was invariably noted and he was brought to book and bidden to mend his ways.

Unlike Wright, who dispensed wisdom to all and sundry at the tea-table, Fitzgerald reserved his lunch-time talk for the hierarchy. And it was an unwritten rule that it was only they who sat at his table. Even they had to be careful because, no matter how eminent they might be, none of them must sit in the seat reserved for the Chief, even when he was away.

Strange as it may seem, this minute attention to diet did not save a high proportion of the older members from gastric troubles, and on one occasion I was the eighth and only intact person at a table seating seven others, all of whom were not only suffering from gastric ulcers but comparing notes on their symptoms in revolting detail.

Recreation also received detailed attention on the same floor. Unless one was a cripple, one was expected to play deck tennis. Whether one was any good at it did not seem to matter. But it was advisable to do so because it brought one's desire to maintain one's health to the notice of the Chief, who participated whenever he could. There was even an annual tournament with a cup for the winners; singles were taboo, they did not encourage the team spirit. As there were only two courts but quite a lot of staff, those not playing could amuse themselves with table tennis. This was considered quite meritorious provided it was interlarded with the occasional bout of the more strenuous game. There was also a billiard table but those who played on it were looked upon as decidely inferior. It was generally considered that their chances of promotion were slender.

The great event in the recreational year was the annual golf tournament. It consisted of a round of golf – usually without bothering about rules or score – followed by a dinner which even non-golfers were expected to attend. Like all Canadian dinners, alcohol could not be served at the meal so that large quantities of rye whisky had to be consumed first. Almost the national drink of Canada, it is cheap, intoxicates quickly and can be mixed with almost anything. But nothing can disguise its awful taste.

The combined effects of this dreadful drink, rich food and unwonted exercise in the open air, tended to make the members of the Connaught Golfing Society, as it was called, so somnolent that anything that went on during the rest of the evening did not matter. But the event was generally considered to be a demonstration for all to see, that whatever might happen elsewhere *mens sana in corpora sano* was certainly practised in the Connaught.

Fitzgerald had other foibles that had an impact on life in the laboratory. Not only so detesting disease that he made its eradication his life's work, he detested noise even more; so much so, that the tap of heels on the hard floors that paved the institution was anathema to him, for which reason every newcomcr was warned to get himself or herself shod with rubber heels before arriving. Loud laughter and, above all, singing would have been the signal for instant dismissal.

Nevertheless, provided one avoided Rabelaisian humour, which he did not like; the making of loud noises; played deck tennis with becoming frequency and golf once a year; and taught preventive medicine in the way he wanted it taught, Fitzgerald was an almost ideal Chief. He was always interested in what one was doing and kept himself up with progress by dropping in about once a week for a chat. He had known most of the pioneers, and although by the time I got to know him he had given up laboratory work, he knew enough about it to sympathize with one's problems. To me he was a very great man and Canada was all the poorer when he died.

When, therefore, I went to work with him, prevention rather than the cure of disease was to be my principal objective. As I have already explained, this consisted for the most part of the prevention of diseases caused by microbes, largely because these were the only diseases that lent themselves to prevention at that time. The techniques employed varied according to the disease and in the way it was transmitted. Those due to microbes that infect the intestinal tract such as cholera, dysentery and typhoid fever, for example, could to a large extent be prevented by due attention to sewage disposal, purification of water supplies and hygiene in the kitchen. Yellow fever and typhus could be prevented by control of the insects that carry them. And smallpox, cholera, plague and rabies could be prevented by making possible victims resistant by the administration of vaccines. But there remained many others whose prevention was still not possible.

Such then, was the position in the mid-1920s. One of the diseases whose prevention was still *sub judice* was diphtheria. There were indications that it could be prevented by immunization, but the preparation used up to that time possessed certain drawbacks which militated against its widespread adoption. A more suitable immunizing agent becoming available about that time, Fitzgerald saw his opportunity and made history by conclusively demonstrating its value. So successful was he that by the time I arrived in Canada, diphtheria had ceased to be the menace it had been for so many years.

I must admit that I had not heard of this before I accompanied the students on the Field Course. I then learned, for the first time, that there had been no deaths from the disease in Toronto since 1934. Even more remarkable was Hamilton, a pleasant town at the western end of Lake Ontario and about 60 miles from Toronto, to which Dr and Mrs Nelles Silverthorne had taken us soon after our arrival. Here there had not been a single case of the disease since 1933 and no deaths since 1930.

Not having taken much interest in diphtheria before I left, I knew very little about the state of affairs in England. But I did know that it was still common; so much so, that when I was attempting to keep one lesson ahead of the twenty students I was instructing during the following winter, I was chagrined to find that in 1935, the year before my departure, there had been 4,337 cases amongst London school children. There had actually been fewer, 3,646 in 1924, the year I qualified; and in the intervening years, the numbers were generally over 5,000.

Having thought before my departure that my country was far ahead of the rest of the world in the practice of preventive medicine, I was naturally taken aback at this demonstration that a nation generally considered to consist of backwoodsmen or prairie farmers had, so to speak, stolen a march on us and succeeded in doing something that we had not even seriously considered. I did not know it then, but I was soon to find out why. Canada had a Fitzgerald, we had not.

Before he took a hand in the proceedings, the only methods employed for the prevention of the disease were to isolate the patient and give contacts diphtheria antitoxin which might protect them for a week or two but not longer. A third procedure was to keep any carriers away from school. These were children who appeared to be perfectly healthy but whose throats harboured virulent diphtheria bacilli. Unfortunately, no one knew how to rid them of their microbes. One of my earliest bacteriological duties at St Mary's had been to deputize for someone who ran a clinic at which these children were given a vaccine in the hope that the bacilli might be induced to leave them. They usually did but not until several months had elapsed, and even then probably because they wanted a change of scenery, for I doubt whether the vaccine played any part in their departure. Not only were such carriers common but they were a nuisance to everyone concerned because they were not allowed to go to school. Their teachers complained that their education suffered, and their parents complained that, as they had to stay at home, they got into mischief. Futile as all this was, it was at that time the only method for the prevention of further cases of the disease that the public health authorities of my country could suggest.

At the very time that I was holding these useless clinics at St Mary's, Fitzgerald was starting his campaign that would soon prevent the disease occurring at all, and in the process rid the community of its carriers. This had become possible because, for a number of technical reasons, diphtheria lends itself to prevention by prophylactic immunization more easily than most forms of bacterial infection. All that is required is to ensure that the antibody known as an antitoxin – which is able to neutralize the toxin or poison produced by the organism – is present in adequate amounts in the circulating blood of potential victims of the disease. To bring this about it is necessary to employ the toxin which is produced when the organism is grown in broth. The microbes are removed by filtration and the clear yellowish fluid constitutes the crude toxin.

If, then, minute doses of this toxin were administered by subcutaneous injection, antitoxin would eventually appear in the blood. But, unfortunately, the toxin is so poisonous that it cannot be used in this way. Even a slight overdose might be fatal. Many attempts were made to get over this difficulty. One of the most successful was to mix the toxin with antitoxin produced in horses. Great care and skill had to be exercised in its preparation; but despite this, Dr W. H. Park in New York had shown, during and after the First World War, that injections of this mixture into children would induce them to produce enough antitoxin to protect themselves against the disease.[66]

Although this showed that diphtheria could be prevented, there were many objections to the use of this method on a large scale. But in 1924 Gustav Ramon, a Frenchman working in the Pasteur Institute in Paris, produced something that was safer, easier to make and therefore cheaper. All that was required was to add a small quantity of formalin to the toxin and incubate the mixture for about a month at 37°C (98·6°F). By that time the poisonous qualities of the toxin had disappeared but, and this is the important point, it still retained its ability to stimulate the formation of antitoxin following its injection. The modified toxin was called anatoxine by Ramon but, because of possible confusion with antitoxin, it is generally known as toxoid.[68]

Fitzgerald heard about the new preparation soon after its

discovery, and went to Paris to investigate it further. He cabled Dr P. J. Moloney, a chemist on his staff, telling him how to make it. Moloney started to do so, and when problems arose he cabled back to Paris for advice about their solution. Despite this expensive and clumsy method of communication, Moloney made what was probably the first toxoid for diphtheria prophylaxis in North America.

It is comparatively easy to make a prophylactic but quite another matter to get it used and even more difficult to get it used properly. And in 1924, nothing was really known about the capabilities of toxoid. If then the Connaught made it and sold it or even gave it to general practitioners, no one would be any the wiser about its value as a prophylactic. If it was to be used at all, better far that it be used in such a way that something could be learned about its abilities to prevent the disease.

It was at this point that Fitzgerald's particular genius began to manifest itself. Tall, slim, quiet, completely master of his emotions and in full possession of all the facts, he never hectored or bullied. He merely suggested, without appearing to do so, a line of attack that not only seemed logical but almost inevitable. Besides Dr Moloney who was already making the toxoid, and his own pupils and colleagues: Dr R. D. Defries, Dr D. T. Fraser, Dr M. D. Orr, Dr Neil McKinnon and Dr Mary Ross, he enlisted the aid of Dr James Roberts, the enthusiastic and energetic Medical Officer of Health of the City of Hamilton, and attacked diphtheria amongst its 150,000 inhabitants.

In 1924, immediately before they started, there had been no less than 400 cases per 100,000 of its population and there had been even more in three out of the four preceding years. But only 3 years later, in 1927, there were only 10 cases per 100,000. In succeeding years the rate continued to fall so much that in 1933 there were no cases at all. Toronto, at that time a city of about 550,000 inhabitants, soon followed suit. There the campaign began in December 1926, and by June 1929 no less than 36,189 children had been immunized or were found not to be in need of it; with, as a result, a 75 per cent reduction in the number of expected cases of diphtheria. And in the year 1931–2, there were only 3 cases amongst those who had been immunized. Of equal importance was the fact that from 1927 to 1932 there were no deaths from diphtheria at all.[23, 61]

With this massive demonstration of the value of immunization as an example, the rest of Ontario and the other Provinces and cities of Canada soon followed suit to such good purpose that by the time I arrived in Toronto in 1936, diphtheria had become a very rare disease over very large areas of Mercator's projection.

This was what was achieved. But in its early stages it was not plain sailing. In the first place a great deal of sales resistance had to be overcome. Mass immunization of this kind was not only a new experience for the inhabitants, but what they had seen of immunization previously cannot have been encouraging. All that they had encountered was vaccination against smallpox, and the administration of typhoid vaccine to the men who had been in the army during the war. Neither were painless or pleasant experiences, and most parents probably anticipated that diphtheria immunization would be much the same.

It was found that much depended on the co-operation of the school-teachers. Many of them knew how much a child's schooling could be delayed by its absence if it was found to be a carrier, and did all they could to persuade parents to consent. Some were less enthusiastic, and one at least was antagonistic because he was a Christian Scientist. But, in one way or another a sufficient number of children were given the new preparation to make the effort worthwhile.

In the second place, great care had to be taken to avoid the general practitioners thinking that the Health Department was attempting to usurp their functions in the community. They were quite prepared to give the toxoid to their patients – provided their patients paid them for doing so. But so high a proportion of the children came from homes that were either unwilling or unable to afford medical treatment at all, or only in the direst emergency, that there would have been very little immunization if it had been left to private enterprise. When, therefore, letters were sent to all parents telling them what was in train they were given three alternatives. The first was that they could have the child immunized by their doctor, the second that it could be done at school for nothing, and the third that they could refuse to have it done at all. A high proportion of the parents of Toronto evidently chose the third alternative because they did not even bother to reply to the letter. But a sufficient number chose the second to enable the investigation to start.

Nor was the immunization itself a simple matter. Since all the children were of school age, 5–14 years old, and diphtheria had been rampant for so long that a high proportion were immune already so that they did not need toxoid, it was necessary to carry out Schick tests to eliminate them. This entailed an injection into the skin of each forearm and its inspection 4 days later. Three more injections at monthly intervals were then necessary.

Since the school medical officers already had enough to do, teams of doctors and nurses had to be hired to do the immunizations. Special arrangements had to be made to carry out bacteriological tests to determine whether any children subsequently suspected of having diphtheria really had the disease, because the clinical diagnosis is not always certain. And, finally, an elaborate organization had to be set up in the School of Hygiene to determine how valuable the new procedure was.

Laborious and time-consuming though the whole business was, it proved that three doses of toxoid would prevent diphtheria, and that the substance was so harmless that none of the children suffered anything resembling the unpleasantness that followed vaccination against smallpox or typhoid fever. It was, in its way, an almost perfect model of how such an investigation should be carried out, and what a boon had come to mankind as a result.

This was already apparent as early as 1930, and one would have thought that every country in the world with any regard for the health of its citizens would have followed suit. Some did. But not Great Britain. The Ministry of Health never went so far as to forbid immunization against diphtheria, but it was less than enthusiastic about it. There were, it is true, certain theoretical objections to this form of immunization but they had already been or were soon shown to be invalid. Whether this was the reason or not, the best that the Ministry of Health could do was to 'recommend' the use of toxoid, which was tantamount to doing nothing.

In consequence of this there were about 60,000 cases of diphtheria every year in England and Wales between 1930 and 1941, so that altogether there must have been well over half-a-million cases of a disease already known to be almost, if not completely, preventable.

In London the situation became almost Gilbertian. The Health Department of the London County Council – which always considered itself to be more advanced than anyone else, and which already had an excellent laboratory producing antitoxin for the treatment of the disease – started about 1937 to plan, and finally opened in 1939, a brand-new, very large and very expensive laboratory in which to make still greater quantities of antitoxin. They no doubt congratulated themselves on their foresight for there were, it is true, no less than 3,656 cases of the disease amongst London school children in 1937, most of whom would have required the antitoxin. But they either forgot or ignored the simple fact that there had been only three cases amongst immunized school children in Toronto as long ago as 1931–2, and which were equally infrequent at the time they started to build the laboratory in which to make the antitoxin to treat cases that need not have occurred at all.

Small wonder that this laboratory became a white elephant at the end of the war. It was given to the Medical Research Council. Amongst the other valuable uses to which that body put it was the provision for me of a scientific home after my retirement, and in which I 're-discovered' penicillin in 1966.

It was not until the blitz arrived in the winter of 1941–2 that the Ministry at last caught up with the times. With a high proportion of the populations of London and the big cities sleeping in air-raid shelters cheek by jowl with the many carriers of the organism known to exist, there was a serious risk of epidemics of the disease. The Ministry accordingly plucked up enough courage to publicize the virtues of diphtheria immunization. The public never hesitated. If toxoid could prevent diphtheria, they wanted it – and soon. But, inefficient to the end, the Ministry had omitted to provide itself with enough toxoid. It had to be imported from America in a hurry. And as had happened in Toronto all of 14 or 15 years before, the disease began to disappear and the carriers with it. It is now almost extinct.

Successful as Fitzgerald and his colleagues had been in defeating diphtheria, there were many other diseases that refused to be dealt with in so cavalier a fashion. By far the most important were those of the respiratory tract such as colds, influenza and pneumonia. Except for the fact that many cases of pneumonia were known to be due to a very distinctive organism called *Diplococcus pneumoniae*, it was not even certain as recently as 1930 what variety of organisms caused most of these infections. But opinion was beginning to harden that many of them were due to viruses.

It was a very long time before it was finally proved that colds are due to viruses but influenza proved more amenable; so much so that when an epidemic of the disease appeared in 1933, Wilson Smith, Christopher Andrewes and Sir Patrick Laidlaw, working in the Mill Hill laboratories of the Medical Research Council, found that if washings from the noses and throats of patients with the disease were instilled into the noses of ferrets, they contracted a disease closely resembling influenza in human beings. If further proof were needed, one of the ferrets was so ill-mannered as to sneeze at a visiting worker who, 48 hours later, went down with typical influenza. Except for the fact that once isolated in the ferret, the virus could cause pneumonia in mice, little more was known about it at the time I arrived in Canada.

It was the study of this virus that was to be my principal activity during the next 10 years. But knowing something of Fitzgerald's history, I was well aware that a great many of the avenues along which research on what was virtually a new virus could have been prosecuted, had better be avoided. It would, for example, have been inadvisable to study its probable shape, size, specific gravity, and chemical composition – all legitimate exercises for a scientist – but more likely to increase his reputation than benefit Mankind. No, this was not what Fitzgerald required of me. He wanted a vaccine or something of a similar nature that would protect human beings against the disease. But he never told me to do it. It was not his habit to tell anyone to do anything. He did not even suggest it. He merely conveyed, in some subtle fashion all of his own, that in the fulness of time, I would produce a prophylactic that would be as successful as that with which he had combated diphtheria.

Unfortunately, I knew as little about virology at the time of my arrival as I did about preventive medicine. In fact, it amounted to no more than what I had read and picked up during a morning spent with Wilson Smith at Mill Hill. It was therefore decreed that I spend a week in New York learning what I could from Dr Thomas Francis at the Rockefeller Institute who was also studying the virus.

In those days a visit to the Rockefeller as it was usually called was something akin to a pilgrimage to Mecca, it was considered to be the holy of holies in the bacteriological world. Few bacteriologists went so far as to prostrate themselves in its direction at sundown but it was said to be peopled by geniuses, inspired for the most part by Dr Oswald T. Avery, and ruled by a Director only slightly less powerful than Allah himself. We had all heard fabulous tales of what went on there: how smoking was forbidden in the lift (so that someone had burnt himself badly by having to conceal a lighted cigarette in his pocket when the Director entered at the last moment); how this same Director, having found Hideyo Noguchi one of the best known of its bacteriologists, with his hat and coat on in the entrance hall during the morning, reprimanded him for arriving late when, in actual fact, the poor fellow was just leaving after spending the night at his bench; still worse was the story that a young Englishman with quite good work to his credit, and who desired to spend a year in the institute, was told that it would be all the better for its reputation if he did not.

Fortunately, I did not encounter the Director, everyone was as helpful as possible and with my virological education completed in this way I returned to Toronto to prepare for an epidemic of the disease that was already starting in Europe and would undoubtedly cross the Atlantic before very long. Ferrets had to be obtained, isolation quarters in which to put them, someone trained to look after them, and all the necessary equipment ordered.

When the epidemic arrived I soon began to lose what friends I had made amongst the staff of the laboratories. Any who were misguided enough to become infected were required to gargle broth and allow the abstraction of blood for the further investigation of their illness. The garglings were instilled into the noses of ferrets. Unfortunately neither my solitary technician Bill Riehm, nor I, had ever handled ferrets before. At first we were frightened out of our wits. But we not only succeeded in avoiding serious mutilation by their teeth, but in keeping them alive. In fact they stood a better chance of survival than we did. For in order to protect ourselves against infection and to avoid transmitting the virus from one ferret to another, we had to encase ourselves in clothing that was neither decorative nor comfortable. For example, we both had to wear masks that covered not only our nose and mouth but our heads as well so that we looked like houris in yashmaks. This nearly stifled us. To add to our discomfort we both wore enormous rubber mackintoshes, large gum-boots and heavy rubber gloves. The whole of this carapace had to be swabbed down with lysol on entering the room, and between each ferret, so that the fumes of cresol added further to our discomfort. It was made even worse by the ether used for anaesthetizing the animals before dropping our friend's garglings on to their noses.

Twice a day thereafter, Bill took the temperatures of the animals by inserting a thermometer into their rectums. How he did it I never knew for I was coward enough to have other engagements at the material times. But done it was. And much to our satisfaction, some of the animals did catch influenza. Few of the young gentlemen and elegantly dressed technicians of the present day, who isolate viruses in tissue cultures in the comfort of their laboratories, have any idea what it meant to be a virologist before the war.

Judge of our chagrin therefore, when I found at the end of the epidemic that, by not far short of superhuman efforts on our part, we had succeeded in isolating the virus from seven out of nine garglings, whereas Francis in New York had done it from no less than sixty specimens. Clearly, we were up against stiff opposition.

Once isolated in the ferret the virus could be transferred to mice, which could be handled in the laboratory and so made life easier. But we were still no nearer to a vaccine for the prevention of the disease. Such a vaccine consists, basically, of a suspension of microbes killed by a suitable method. For obvious reasons foreign substances should not be present. This is not difficult to ensure when the vaccine consists of microbes that will grow on culture media. But viruses will not grow in this way; they will only grow in living cells. And when the only cells in which they grow are in the lungs of ferrets or mice, it follows that if they are ground up with sand and saline to provide a suspension of virus particles, there will be a great deal too much ferret or mouse tissue in the mixture as well. One cannot inject anything like this into human beings without courting a disaster sooner or later.

There was, however, another possibility. Long before coming to Canada, while I was still at Queen Charlotte's, a patient had been admitted who was seriously ill with influenza. Although she had just had a baby she was not suffering from puerperal fever. Colebrook was away at the time engaged on his annual winter sport pilgrimage to Switzerland and I was in charge of the patients. Reasoning that if we gave her serum from someone who had just had influenza it might contain antibodies that would neutralize her virus and so cure her, I set about finding a suitable donor. Fortunately Dr Davies, a friend of Dora Colebrook's, had just recovered from the disease and allowed us to take some of her blood. We gave the patient 2 c.c. of the serum that afternoon when she was rapidly becoming so seriously ill that it was beginning to be doubtful whether she would last the night. At 10.00 p.m. they phoned to say she was much better. Still very nervous about the whole business, I suggested another 2 c.c. of the serum. Next morning she was sitting up in bed reading the newspaper, so for good measure we gave her 5 c.c. She made a completely uninterrupted recovery, and I invariably succeeded in infuriating everybody by saying that until the sulphonamides appeared in 1935 she was the only patient at Queen Charlotte's we could claim to have actually cured.

This was in 1933, and about the time the virus was being discovered not far away at Mill Hill. Why not infect ferrets with the virus, allow them to recover, remove their blood and use it for the treatment or even the prevention of cases of the disease? The serum could, if necessary, be purified so that it need be no more dangerous than that of horses which was used for the prevention of tetanus.

We then embarked on a long series of experiments that showed it was possible to protect mice against infection in this way. But when we tried to protect ferrets, whose disease resembles that of human beings more closely, all we succeeded in doing was to make them worse. We never found out why, but the use of ferret serum is not one of my contributions to the welfare of the human race.

About the time that the remedial qualities of convalescent ferret serum had finally become discredited, another and more elegant source of virus became available. This was the allantoic fluid in the developing fertile egg of a barnyard fowl. The technical details of its production do not matter but the virus was first injected into the egg through a hole made in the shell, so that the virus could grow in the cells of the chorioallantoic membrane which lies inside the shell. When produced, the virus appears in quite large amounts in the allantoic fluid inside the membrane. Since the fluid is in all essentials the urine of the developing embryo, it contains urates and a little protein. Except for this it was a much cleaner source of virus than the soups we had previously employed. Relatively large amounts of the fluid could easily be obtained by suction.

This playing about with eggs gave us a method for the detection of the virus that we had not anticipated. For one day Dr Laurella McClelland observed that if the virus was present in the allantoic fluid, any red cells from vessesls in the chorioallantoic membrane that had been ruptured while taking the fluid, ran together into clumps, or, in bacteriological language, agglutinated. If there was no virus in the egg this did not occur, and the escaped blood became evenly distributed in the fluid.

This enabled us to tell at a glance whether or not the virus had grown in the eggs. It was obviously a discovery of considerable importance.

For the next few weeks we did little else but study it. We soon found that what occurred is that a virus particle attaches itself to the surface of a red cell and remains stuck to it. Another red cell then becomes attached to the other side of the virus particle. More virus particles attached to the cells attract more red cells, so that in time large, clearly visible masses of red cells with attached virus are obtained, This was one of the first occasions on which the phenomenon we now know as haemagglutination was observed.

This in itself was important, but even more so was the fact that if a serum containing neutralizing antibody had previously been added to the virus, the virus no longer adhered to the red cells. There was no agglutination. We had discovered not only a method of detecting the virus without recourse to the expensive and time-consuming animal tests with mice that had hitherto been essential, but also a method for measuring antibodies that took only an hour or so.[62]

Within a week or so of this discovery, Dr Hirst of New York published a paper in *Science* reporting very similar findings. Almost overnight, this changed virology from an exercise in the management of whole zoos of animals into something resembling an exact science.

Using the virus in allantoic fluid inactivated by formalin as a vaccine, and our new method of detecting and measuring antibodies, we then injected a number of our friends and colleagues with the vaccine and studied the antibodies they produced. They increased in amount but not as much as was desirable if they were to be protected against infection. Evidently not enough virus was present in the fluid.

As we could not persuade the egg to produce more, we would have to concentrate the fluid in some way. For a time this problem seemed insoluble. But one day I was sitting in the laboratory talking to Dr McLelland when I happened to notice a large bottle of allantoic fluid that had been frozen solid and was standing on the bench. By now it had melted and there was a large white mass at the bottom of the bottle with, above it, a perfectly clear supernatant. I knew that if the bottle was shaken and warmed, the precipitate would go into solution. But instead of doing this, the clear fluid was withdrawn very carefully and the precipitate shaken up with what remained of the fluid. Using the new method of titration, we soon found that most of the virus had come down in the precipitate.

The white paste produced in this way could not be used for the immunization of human beings. We then embarked on a long series of experiments to find how to elute the virus, as the chemists express it, from the solid materials to which it was evidently attached. This proved to be surprisingly easy. Treatment with buffer solutions at different pH's or isinglass solution gave us a water clear solution that could be freeze-dried and kept indefinitely. Would this concentrated vaccine protect human beings against influenza?[49]

During the autumn of 1942 we transformed ourselves into a miniature factory for the manufacture of vaccine prepared in this way. To simplify matters we confined ourselves to influenza A virus. An epidemic of influenza caused by this virus was expected in the early months of 1943, so we enlisted the aid of the university health departments in Vancouver, Edmonton and Winnipeg while we ourselves gave it to our class in Toronto. We immunized 262 persons in this way and gave a control vaccine to another 259. We then sat back and waited for the epidemic to materialize. It did. But unfortunately, instead of influenza A, influenza B turned up. Naturally our vaccine did not protect against this form of the disease. We were back where we started.

By the time we had worked all this out, the summer of 1943 had arrived. When we should have been preparing for the epidemic that did, a year late, make its appearance in the autumn and winter of 1943–4, I was engaged on other and more useful pursuits, concerning the manufacture of penicillin, that have been related in the preceding chapter. Research on influenza vaccines went into hibernation during that winter.

When the summer of 1944 arrived, another vaccine had made its appearance. It had been sponsored by my friend Francis. This too was a concentrated vaccine, but made by a different process. When withdrawing the allantoic fluid from the eggs, blood vessels in the chorioallantoic membrane were purposely ruptured. The virus attached itself to the cells which settled to the bottom of the bottle. The clear fluid above was removed, saline added to the cells and the mixture incubated at 37°C (98·6°F) for 2½ hours by which time the virus had left the red cells and gone into suspension again into the saline. The red cells were removed by centrifugation, and formalin added to the saline suspension, in this way completing its preparation.

This vaccine had been used for the immunization of no less than 6,263 persons during the preceding winter, of whom 138 got influenza. It was therefore not completely protective. But of 6,211 controls, 442 became infected. There was something to be said for the vaccine. But not much.[14]

Despite this, Washington ordered large quantities from manufacturers in the United States. Unfortunately for me, it had become a more or less unwritten rule by this time that whatever Washington did, Ottawa did too. It did, and required us to make 200,000 doses. In the process we used 3,000 fertile eggs a day for the best part of 6 months. They were processed on an assembly line using a moving belt in a darkened room, the girls who were doing it wearing gloves all the time. How they stood it I never knew. This was carried out at the farm while we in the city completed the process. Ottawa duly received its 200,000 doses and never was I more thankful than when it was all over.

I never bothered to find out what happened to the vaccine. I had too little faith in it. I suspect it was never used. At all events, that made in the United States at the same time was found to be useless. Those who had received it were not immune to the virus when it made its next appearance in 1947. The virus had cheated. It had so altered its chemical constitution in the interval that it resisted the antibodies.

It was in this state of disillusionment that I went to Cambridge in the summer of 1948 to attend a meeting of the British Medical Association, and tell an audience that saw an egg only about once a month that it would be better to eat eggs rather than use them for the manufacture of influenza vaccine. They did, at least contain vitamins.

I accordingly took little interest in the disease or possible vaccines for its prevention until 1961, when I visited Toronto for the first time since my departure 15 years previously. Much to my surprise I learned from Dr J. K. W. Ferguson, who by that time had become Director of the Connaught, that in 1957 they had resuscitated the method we had evolved in 1942 for the production of a vaccine by freezing and thawing and that it had actually been used in Canada. Needless to say I was gratified by this information, if only because it showed that I had not been forgotten, but still more because it relieved my mind on one point. I had not, as I had thought, all those years, failed Fitzgerald when he charged me with the production of a prophylactic for influenza. And although it was never used on any scale until 1957, 17 years after his death, it was, in a sense, his vaccine. I had, after all, done what he expected of me.

Nevertheless, neither this vaccine nor any of the others that have so far been evolved, can be considered major triumphs in the combating of influenza. A proportion of those who receive them, but by no means all, may be protected. There is, accordingly, little justification for their widespread use at the present time.

Much more successful was immunization against tetanus, another major Connaught activity before and during the war. Toxoid, made in much the same way as that used for the prevention of diphtheria was employed for this purpose. I was not directly concerned with its production but was frequently called upon to help Dr P. A. T. Sneath and Dr D. T. Fraser, one of the best friends I have ever had, when they had to abstract blood from the volunteers in whom they were testing it. But thanks to immunization with this toxoid, the disease which had been a comparatively common complication of wounds sustained in all previous wars, was almost unknown during the Second World War.

A second common complication of warfare is typhus. Being transmitted by lice, it is particularly liable to occur in destitute and homeless families in revolutions or among soldiers on campaigns who cannot wash themselves or their clothing. A vaccine for the prevention of this disease was also evolved during the early stages of the war. It was made, like that used for influenza, in fertile eggs. But it was much more successful; so successful that enormous quantities were made by Dr James Craigie with whom I used to play table tennis before the war. But because the microbes that cause the disease are amongst the most dangerous in existence, he spent most of the war in purdah in a building at the farm into which none of us were allowed, or wanted, to penetrate. There was, in consequence, no more table tennis and in any event post-luncheon recreation had to stop. It took up space needed for other things. Even the billiard table went into store.

When at long last the war ended with VJ day in the summer of 1945, I could say that, having worked in the Inoculation Department and Queen Charlotte's Hospital, I knew all about the treatment of bacterial infections, and my 10 years at the Connaught Laboratories had instructed me how to prevent them. It was high time I put all this hard-won knowledge to some use. The upshot of it all was that I was ordered to present myself at the Senate House of the University of London on the afternoon of July 12, 1946.

Chapter 11

The Metamorphosis of Medicine

The end of June 1946 found me on an ex-banana boat which was loading sides of bacon in one of the docks in Montreal. After an uneventful voyage I arrived at the Royal Albert Dock in the early hours of July 12, and had just enough time to present myself at the University of London for the interview. It ended in my being appointed to the newly established Chair of Bacteriology in the University at St Thomas's Hospital Medical School.

Except for the fact that the post was permanent, the prospect was not encouraging. Much of the hospital was derelict, having received several direct hits probably meant for Downing Street not far away. Only one ward was in action, most of the patients and clinical students being still at Hydestile near Godalming in in Surrey, 40 miles away.

The Medical School had escaped serious damage, but most of the library books were still away in the country and the Pathological Museum was a shambles. Nearly all the specimens had survived because they had been buried before the bombing started, but their disinterment, identification and remounting took two technicians the best part of 2 years. Being a newly created department, there was nowhere to put me and I had to make do with a cold draughty barn of a place in the hospital, whose roof leaked so much that waterproof covers had to be placed over electrical apparatus whenever rain was expected. Its entire stock of equipment consisted of one ancient autoclave, an oven long past its prime, an incubator, a dozen petri dishes whose lids did not fit, the same number of pipettes, most of them broken, and two microscopes that had seen better days. The staff consisted of Dr T. Martin, an almost untrained technician, and a succession of secretaries none of whom stayed for more than a week or so and some, having accepted the appointment, never turned up at all.

Strange as it may seem, within 18 months I had acquired by purchase, gift or petty larceny, most of the apparatus and materials with which to start research; a staff that seemed likely to stay, and a pre-fab building was going up for me on the roof of the medical school with one of the fairest views in London. And 9 months later we collected enough alcohol and cigarettes to entertain most of the bacteriological talent of London.

I do not propose to describe my activities during the 18 years I spent in this eyrie. They were too multifarious. But it was not very long before I became aware that medicine was very different from what it had been in my student days and, in fact, until the outbreak of the war. The atmosphere of a large teaching hospital such as St Thomas's was certainly very different. There were several reasons for this. One was that for all practical purposes all the hospitals had been nationalized at the outbreak of the war, and the coming of the National Health Service in 1948 which took them over was merely the final stage in the process. This absolved them from the necessity to beg for money to enable them to exist at all. But it also gave them access to the apparently bottomless cornucopia in Whitehall from which the Socialist Government dispensed riches undreamed of by hospital administrators before the war. One result was that there was a pullulation of young men in the guise of registrars and house officers in every hospital. They brought an enthusiasm previously unknown which replaced the *laissez faire* of the years before the war. Many of them were making real attempts to prevent, cure, or at the very least study disease. They had learned what research could do. In fact, their survival at all was partly due to research by the physicists that had led to radar, which saved the country in the summer of 1940. And all of them knew that penicillin was the fruit of research.

What is more, medical research had become respectable and

was no longer a spare time hobby for slightly abnormal pathologists, or something to occupy the time of men endowed with private means. It could now be a career in itself, with an adequate salary and pension met from the vast sums of money that now became available from government departments, the Medical Research Council, the universities and the trusts set up by societies interested in particular diseases. But as research workers are born, not made, and the proportion of the population with the necessary talents did not rise in step with the money available to pay them, it not only became difficult to find suitable individuals but much of the research that emerged was mediocre at best. This was perhaps inevitable but a great deal of very useful and important work was done.

Another stimulant to do research was that as a result of a whole series of technological advances and discoveries made by pharmacologists, physiologists, anatomists and bacteriologists a great many diseases were becoming preventable, curable or amenable to study. Almost every facet of medicine was affected in this way. Even so unpromising a subject as psychiatry was caught up in the march of progress. At one time, its devotees had been generally credited with spending most of their time in debating whether or not to put such and such a patient in a padded cell; they were now using shock therapy and drugs like tranquilizers to such good purpose that lunatics were being cured and asylums began to call themselves mental hospitals. The anaesthetists, too, were given new life. Better anaesthetics and measures for the prevention and relief of shock enabled them to play a real part in the operating theatre instead of gossiping with the surgeon and pouring ether on to a mask. And the surgeon himself not only peered into portions of the human anatomy previously denied him, but actually carried out experiments on animals to find out how to do it.

In this way practically every hospital, and teaching hospitals most of all, became hives of industry after the war. And it was not very long before it became difficult to find somewhere to put all the seekers after medical truths. Any accommodation, no matter how small, was immediately snapped up. One of my friends specialized in the detection of redundant lavatories and stair cupboards, and when no one was looking, converted them into laboratories. A flat roof was a possession beyond price because a hut could be put on it even though mountaineering ability and a head for heights were required to get to it. Safer of approach but equally desirable were lawns and gardens; they too sprouted huts and even caravans.

How very different all this was from what it had been before the war. And no wonder that so much disease was prevented or cured when all this thought and effort were given to it in this way. But for all that, by far the most spectacular advances were made in combating diseases caused by microbes. I have already described the early stages of this process, but it gathered momentum in no uncertain fashion as soon as the value of penicillin was established. The mere fact that a mould could evidently produce a useful antibiotic prompted drug firms and research institutes to search for other moulds producing similar substances but which would act on species of microbes unaffected by penicillin. Almost every source of moulds the world over was ransacked in search of them. The soil proved to be the most profitable and many were found in this way.

The first to be discovered was streptomycin. Found in September 1943 by Dr Selman A. Waksman, a distinguished soil microbiologist, its value for the treatment of tuberculosis was still unknown when, shortly afterwards, I met him in Toronto. (He was much more elated by the news of the liberation of his native Kiev by the Russians on the day of his arrival.) Despite its tendency to cause dizziness and even deafness which, for a time, made it doubtful whether it should be used at all, it has proved of such extraordinary value for the treatment of all forms of tuberculosis that patients detected early enough need not even stay in hospital; a far cry from the year or more that had previously been essential.

In 1947 came chloramphenicol, another antibiotic whose adoption was imperilled by effects it might have on patients receiving it, in this instance degeneration of the blood-forming cells in the bone marrow. But so long as it is used wisely, it is still first choice for the treatment of typhoid and typhus fevers. Aureomycin was introduced at the same time, and terramycin in

1950, two more so-called broad-spectrum antibiotics because they act on a wide variety of bacterial species. With the antibiotics so far mentioned, most of the bacteria that cause human infections can generally be controlled.

Other species of organisms that have never been sensitive to any of these antibiotics required special consideration. One was *Pseudomonas pyocyanea*. It only seldom causes infection, and then usually of wounds or the urinary tract. An antibiotic called polymixin which is somewhat unusual in being produced by a bacillus and not a mould, was found to be invaluable for the treatment of such infections. The fungi, too, required their own private antibiotics, nystatin first employed in 1950, griseofulvin in 1959 and amphotericin B as recently as 1962.

Another series of antibiotics too numerous to mention individually, also made their appearance when strains of staphylococci resistant to penicillin became rampant in our hospitals. These too have proved to be invaluable, particularly for the treatment of the infections that may follow operations.

While this was in train, the chemists found that by altering the molecule of penicillin they could produce the so-called semi-synthetic penicillins that have their own particular values. One is ability to resist the acid in the stomach so that such a penicillin can be taken by mouth instead of its having to be injected. Another is ampicillin, of great value for the treatment of infections by intestinal organisms, and a third, methicillin, for the treatment of infections by penicillin-resistant staphylococci.

While antibiotic after antibiotic was being discovered, the chemists produced a whole series of synthetic compounds that have nothing to do with them. The sulphones for example, discovered as early as 1942, have now become the standard treatment for leprosy. Two more, *para*-aminosalycilic acid and isoniazid, form part of the treatment for tuberculosis. Lastly, there are several compounds employed for the treatment of urinary infections, the most recent being nitrofurantoin and nalidixic acid.

As a result of all this activity, there are very few infections caused by microbes that cannot be controlled if not actually cured by one or other of these substances. The viruses, on the other hand, have so far proved resistant. They still cause such diseases as colds, influenza and measles. But although the antibiotics may have no effect on the disease itself, they still have a part to play in their treatment because, under certain circumstances, bacteria may cause secondary infections that are more important than the virus infection itself. Because of this, the bronchopneumonia that may kill a patient with measles or influenza can frequently be controlled if treated with a suitable antibiotic.

If nothing more than this had occurred, it would still have been a major revolution, but the number of diseases that could be prevented from occurring at all steadily increased as the years went by. Prior to the appearance of the new chemotherapy in 1935, such infectious diseases as enteric, cholera and dysentery had become extremely unusual as a result of the sanitary revolution in the nineteenth century. Other measures such as the pasteurization of milk were followed by a considerable reduction in bone and joint tuberculosis; control of mosquitoes could prevent yellow fever, and maritime quarantine: smallpox, plague and cholera.

These measures did no more than hinder or prevent the travels of the microbes and viruses from their sources to potential victims. Much more successful were those that rendered these victims resistant to infection. Smallpox, rabies, plague, typhoid fever and cholera had already become preventable by some form of immunization before the First World War ended. During the 1920s diphtheria was added to the list. About the time the new chemotherapy was being evolved, yellow fever ceased to be the hazard of travel it had once been in half the African continent. Two more vaccines, those protecting against tetanus and typhus, proved their value during the Second World War. Shortly after it, B.C.G. vaccination for the prevention of tuberculosis won its spurs amongst the homeless and destitute populations that the war left in Europe. Then came a vaccine preventing whooping cough. And when antibiotics such as penicillin and streptomycin were found to prevent bacterial contamination so successfully, large scale tissue culture became possible with vaccines for the prevention of poliomyelitis and, more recently, measles.[65]

Almost as astonishing as the advances themselves was the speed with which they were introduced into medicine. Starting in 1946 when penicillin first became easy to obtain, the process was virtually completed in only 5 years. Practically all the antibiotics, synthetic chemicals and prophylactic vaccines to bring it about had been discovered and were already in use before 1951. Those introduced since then have filled gaps or are improvements on those already in use. But it was in those 5 years that microbes ceased to be the menace they had been from the time of Man's evolution half-a-million years ago.

Because of all this, it is now difficult to be seriously ill with an infection and very nearly impossible to die of it. And yet, how few realize the magnitude of this change in our relationship with microbes. Before the new chemotherapy and prophylactic vaccines, fully a third of all the deaths that occurred during the best years of life, that is before the age of 45, and a half and even even more in the childhood years of 1–5, were due to the attentions of microbes and particularly those that cause diphtheria, whooping cough, tuberculosis and measles. But now all these diseases can be prevented by vaccines, and even if the disease actually occurs it can either be cured at once or its worst effects staved off.

Many diseases still cannot be prevented. But they can be treated very effectively; pneumonia and scarlet fever are examples. Infections less likely to be fatal such as boils and carbuncles, skin infections of all kinds, urinary infections, syphilis and gonorrhoea, can now be cut short in days or weeks.

Although I myself had done little, if anything, to bring this about, it was in the hope that something of this nature would eventually transpire that I had become a bacteriologist; I never anticipated the magnitude of the change or the speed with which it would come. I certainly never thought that the type of medical practice I knew as a child or in the hospitals I attended as a student would alter so profoundly.

The optimism and bottles of medicine that sufficed for my father's patients would no longer be adequate for those he visited today. They now demand antibiotics for even the most trivial infections. And so the doctor has to carry syringes round

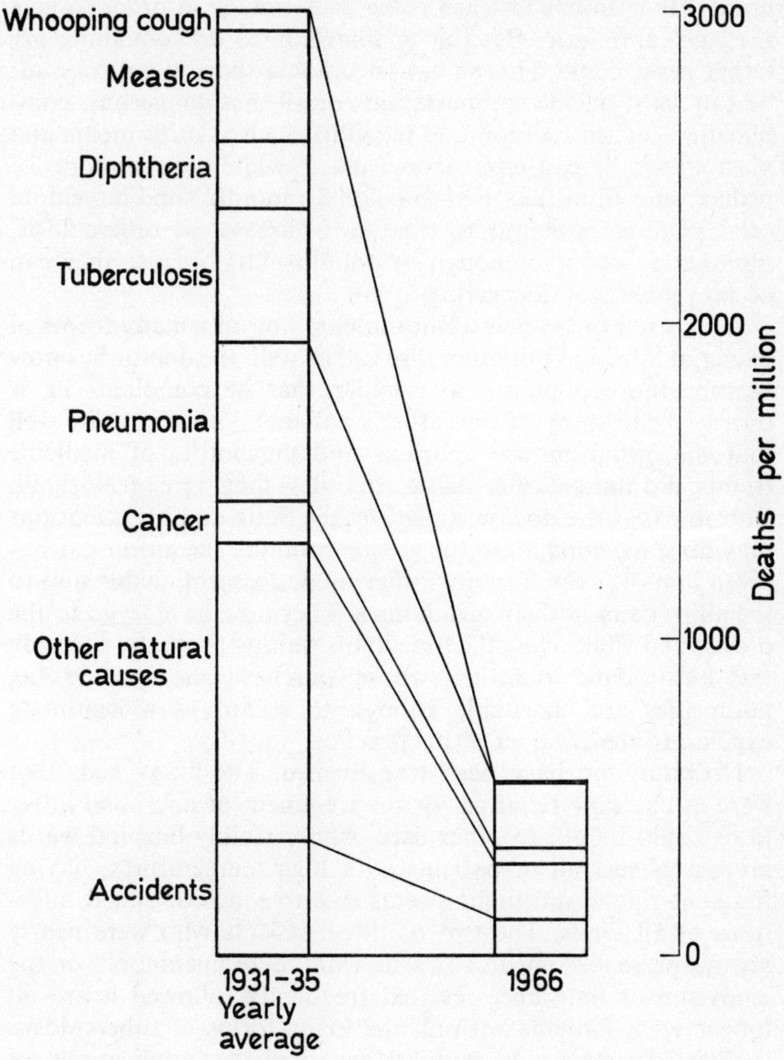

Fig. 3. Comparison between the death rates in early childhood before and after the introduction of the new chemotherapy.

with him – and learn how to sterilize them before he leaves home. He even has to learn some bacteriology in order to give the right antibiotic. But this enables him to do something my father never could. He can cut pneumonia short in a day or so; he can ward off the common, but for all that dangerous, complications of scarlet fever and tonsillitis such as otitis media and mastoiditis; he can cure or at least alleviate the symptoms of urinary infections that used to go on for months; and he seldom sees, let alone attempts to treat such diseases as tuberculosis, diphtheria, whooping cough or poliomyelitis because they can be prevented from occurring at all.

As a result of his new ability to cure not only many forms of bacterial infection but other diseases as well, the doctor has now become more popular; so popular that he complains he is overworked. Many of my father's patients, knowing quite well that the optimism was spurious and the bottles of medicine frauds, did not seek his assistance unless they were seriously ill. But now that the doctor is paid by the State and his attentions may do some good, even the greater mobility the motor-car has given him over the trap my father used, does not enable him to see all of them in their own homes. They now have to go to the doctor and while away the time in his waiting room, by perusing the out-of-date literature whose purchase the income tax authorities are charitable enough to regard as a legitimate expense in the conduct of his practice.

Hospitals too have been transformed. The many beds that were at one time required for the treatment of microbial infections could be put to other uses. And certainly hospital wards are no longer full of patients with high temperatures, having frequent rigors and night sweats due to long-continued infections of all kinds. The two or three patients who were nearly always present in medical wards with acute pneumonia or the empyema or lung abcesses that frequently followed it are no longer seen. Patients with all the many forms of tuberculosis, the tertiary stages of syphilis, the cardiac complications of rheumatic fever, osteomyelitis, erysipelas, deep abcesses, cellulitis, carbuncles, meningitis, otitis media and mastoiditis have become increasingly unusual. Compound fractures still become infected and patients with appendicitis or acute peritonitis still appear in the wards, but with an antibiotic to help them they are seldom in danger and generally recover quickly.

Hospitals for children have, if anything, been affected even more. A much higher proportion of their patients used to occupy their beds because of the attentions of microbes. But with the new control that is possible over them, whole wards have sometimes had to be closed for want of patients to fill them.

The most heavily hit have been the special hospitals which had a vested interest in microbes because their very existence depended on them. One of the first to become redundant in this was the Isolation Block at Queen Charlotte's, which had already become a haven for almoners and physiotherapists by the time I arrived back in England. But it was not very long before others found themselves short of patients. The rapid disappearance of diphtheria and the new ability to prevent the more serious complications of measles and scarlet fever, and before very long the reduction in the number of cases of whooping cough, resulted in some of the previously over-populated isolation hospitals having to find other spheres of activity. One, that in Lawn Road, Hampstead, where many of our puerperal fever patients were at one time treated, has now risen to aristocracy in the social scale of hospitals. It has become a teaching hospital with students of the Royal Free Hospital walking its wards.

Hospitals that specialized in certain forms of disease were not immune. Queen Mary's at Carshalton had, at one time, been almost the world centre for the treatment of bone and joint tuberculosis under Dr Pugh; following the decline in this disease before and during the war the hospital found itself harbouring large numbers of children with rheumatic fever or the damaged hearts that were so common a sequel. But with the decline in streptococcal infections that gave rise to this disease, it had to find other uses for its beds, most of which had nothing to do with microbes. The rapid disappearance of pulmonary tuberculosis and the ease with which it could be treated at home, was inevitably followed by sanatoria having to adapt themselves to the treatment of quite different illnesses. Even mental hospitals were affected, for the many beds once occupied by patients with the neurological manifestations of syphilis were no longer needed for that purpose.

If, as a young man, I had never anticipated the kaleidoscopic changes that would come to medicine, still less did I imagine that within my own lifetime the new control over microbes would cause anxiety about the future of the human race. For it is now exhibiting an unprecedented ability to survive; so much so that children who previously would have died of malnutrition, scarlet fever or diphtheria now reach puberty and start to have children of their own. And the middle-aged man who, 40 years ago, would have died of pneumonia, now escapes to become a burden to his family until he is 80 or even more. And when all this happens within a few years, the population begins to increase at an alarming rate which is best expressed in the words of Prof. Hamid Ali Khan, 'all over the world populations are rising rapidly and no country, young or old, large or small, developed or developing, whether inhabited by coloured people or white, can escape the ravages of this phenomenal population growth'.[46]

What the ultimate effect will be can only be guessed but it is bound to be unpleasant and will certainly involve difficulties in finding enough food, water, minerals and even sleeping room to cope with the inexorable rise in the population of the world that seems almost certain to occur. Thus, despite what the humanitarians may say, it might have been better if bacteriologists and departments of hygiene and preventive medicine in the universities had been rather less active in their desire to eradicate disease and the public health officials who aided and abetted them had been rather more leisurely in the application of their researches. For the end result is that between them, like the physicists who in spite of themselves have let loose the horror of the atomic bomb on the world, they have started a train that may lead to a population explosion that could be quite as important in the history of the world as that at Hiroshima.

Nevertheless, whenever I visited Fleming after my return to England, I always found it very difficult to get used to the idea that he had played so notable a part in bringing this about. It would be impossible to imagine anyone less like a revolutionary, He did not look like one, nor did he talk like one. He did not even behave like one. He was not, for example, guarded by a secretary to keep odd callers at bay. If he had a secretary, she was concealed somewhere else. Nor did he possess an office in which to conceal himself. But he had a laboratory which, as laboratories go, had little to commend it. Its door was perpetually open so that one merely walked in and talked while he fiddled at the bench inventing new techniques or playing with new instruments such as a phase contrast microscope some kindly soul had given him.

It was probably because I saw so much of him in this way that he was instrumental in getting me appointed as the representative of the University of London on the Council of the Wright–Fleming Institute in 1952. And so the wheel had turned full circle and I took my place along with Fleming and Freeman on the governing body of the laboratory I had entered as a raw beginner in 1925. It was the proudest moment of my life.

Early in 1955 Fleming retired, and began to prepare for a long lecture tour he was to make in the Middle East later in the year. And some time during January he asked my wife, son and me to dine with him and Lady Fleming at his flat in Danvers Street. He was as active and as well as ever, delighted with a new camera someone had given him and showing us superb slides of his garden in Suffolk.

It was the last time I saw him, for in March he died suddenly. A few days later we all went to his funeral in St Paul's Cathedral. And so the little, shy, almost inarticulate Scot we all loved so much was the first bacteriologist to take his place beside Nelson, Wellington and Wren. I very much doubt whether he had ever imagined for a moment that such an honour would come to him. And if he had been told that it undoubtedly would, his reaction would have been to turn his head, look one straight in the eye for a moment, tell one not to be ridiculous, and carry on with the experiment. For to Fleming it was the experiment that mattered most, more even than a resting place in the crypt of St Paul's Cathedral.

SOURCES

No attempt has been made to draw up a complete bibliography; it would require a great many pages. I have accordingly confined myself to the more important publications and my sources of information on controversial matters.

1 Abraham, E. P., Chain, C., Fletcher, C. M., Florey, H. W., Gardner, A. D., Heatley, N. G. & Jennings, M. A., 'Further observations on penicillin', *Lancet*, **ii,** 177, 1941

2 Allison, V. D, 'Sir Alexander Fleming, 1881–1955', *J. Gen. Microbiol.*, **14,** 1, 1956

3 Baldry, P. E, *The Battle against Bacteria,* Cambridge University Press, 1965

4 Bigger, J. W., Boland, C. R. & O'Meara, R. A. Q., 'Variant colonies of *Staphylococcus aureus*', *J. Path. Bact.*, **30,** 261, 1927

5 Chain, E., Florey, H. W., Gardner, A. D., Heatley, N. G., Jennings, M. A., Orr-Ewing, J. & Sanders, A. G., 'Penicillin as a chemotherapeutic agent', *Lancet*, **ii**, 226, 1940

6 Clutterbuck, P. W., Lovell, R. & Raistrick, H., 'The formation from glucose by members of the *Penicillium chrysogenum* series of a pigment, an alkali soluble protein and penicillin—the antibacterial substance of Fleming', *Biochem. Jour.*, **26,** 1907, 1932

7 Coghill, R. G. & Koch R. S., 'Penicillin—a wartime accomplishment', *Chem. and Engin. News,* **23,** 2310, 1945

8 Colebrook, D. C., 'The source of infection in puerperal fever due to haemolytic streptococci', *Med. Res. Coucn. Spec. Rep.*, No. 205, London, H.M.S.O., 1935

9 Colebrook, L., 'A study of some organic arsenical compounds with a view to their use in certain streptococcal infections', *Med. Res. Counc. Spec. Rep.*, No. 119, London, H.M.S.O., 1928

10 Colebrook, L., *Almroth Wright*, London, William Heinemann, 1954

11 Colebrook, L., 'Alexander Fleming, 1881–1955', *Biographical Memoirs of Fellows of the Royal Society*, **2,** 117, 1956

12 Colebrook, L., 'Gerhard Domagk, 1895–1964', *Biographical Memoirs of Fellows of the Royal Society*, **10,** 39, 1964

13 Colebrook, L and Kenny, M., 'Treatment of human puerperal infections and of experimental infections in mice with Prontosil', *Lancet*, **i,** 1279, 1936

14 Commission on Influenza, 'A clinical evaluation of vaccination against

influenza', *J. Amer. Med. Assoc.*, **124,** 982, 1944
15 Cope, V. Z., *Almroth Wright: Founder of Modern Vaccine Therapy*, London, Thomas Nelson, 1966
16 Craddock, S. R., Private communication
17 Cruickshank, R., 'Alexander Fleming, 6th August, 1881–11th March, 1955', *J. Path. Bact.*, **72,** 697, 1956
18 Dale, H. H., in 'Sir Alexander Fleming, M.D., D.Sc., F.R.C.P., F.R.C.S., F.R.S.', *Brit. Med. Jour.*, **i,** 732 and 795, 1955
19 Defries, R. D., *The First Forty Years, 1914–55*, Connaught Medical Research Laboratories, Toronto, University of Toronto Press, 1968
20 Domagk, G., 'Ein Beitrag zur Chemotherapie der bacteriellen Infektionen', *Deut. Med. Woch.*, **61,** 250, 1935
21 Domagk, G. & Hegler, C., *Chemotherapie bakterieller Infektionen*, Leipzig, Von S. Hirzel, 1944
22 Ehrlich, P., 'Chemotherapeutics; scientific principles, methods and results', *Lancet*, **ii,** 445, 1913
23 Fitzgerald, J. G., Fraser, D. T., McKinnon, N. E. & Ross, M. A., 'Diphtheria—a preventable disease', *Lancet*, **i,** 391, 1938.
24 Fleming, A., 'On the antibacterial action of cultures of a *Penicillium* with special reference to their use for the isolation of B. influenzae', *Brit. J. Exp. Path.*, **10,** 226, 1929
25 Fleming, A., 'Some problems in the use of antiseptics', *Brit. Dent. Jour.*, **52,** 105, 1931
26 Fleming, A., 'The intravenous use of germicides', *Proc. Roy. Soc. Med.*, **24,** 808, 1931
27 Fleming, A., 'On the specific antibacterial properties of penicillin and potassium tellurite incorporating a method of demonstrating some bacterial antagonisms', *J. Path. Bact.*, **35,** 831, 1932
28 Fleming, A., 'Lysozyme', *Proc. Roy. Soc. Med.*, **26,** 1, 1932
29 Fleming, A., 'Serum and vaccine therapy in combination with sulphanilamide or M and B 693', *Proc. Roy. Soc. Med.*, **32,** 911, 1939
30 Fleming, A., 'The effect of antiseptics on wounds', *Proc. Roy. Soc. Med.*, **33,** 487, 1940
31 Fleming, A., 'Antiseptics and chemotherapy', *Proc. Roy. Soc. Med.*, **33,** 127, 1940
32 Fleming, A., 'Chemotherapy and wound infection', *Proc. Roy. Soc. Med.*, **34,** 342, 1941
33 Fleming, A., 'The discovery of penicillin', *Brit. med. Bull.*, **2,** 4, 1944
34 Fleming, A., The Harben Lectures: 'Penicillin, its discovery, development and uses in the fields of medicine and surgery', *J. Roy. Inst. Pub. Health and Hyg.*, **8,** 36, 63, 93, 1945
35 Fleming, A., 'Antiseptics old and new', *Proc. Staff Meetings, Mayo Clinic.*, **21,** 65, 1946
36 Fleming, A., *Nobel Lecture on Penicillin*, Kungl Boktrichereit, P. A. Stockholm, Norstedt & Soner, 1947

37 Fleming, A. & Porteous, A. B., 'The streptococcal infections of septic wounds at a base hospital', *Lancet*, **i**, 19, 1919
38 Florey, H. W., 'Penicillin: a survey', *Brit. Med. Jour.*, **ii**, 169, 1944
39 Florey, H. W. & Cairns, H., 'The treatment of war wounds with penicillin' *Bull. War. Med.* **4**, 319, 1944
40 Florey, H. W., Chain, E., Heatley, N. G., Jennings, M. A., Sanders, A. G., Abraham, E. P. & Florey, M. E., *Antibiotics*, London, Oxford University Press, 1949
41 Florey, M. E. & Florey, H. W., 'Local and general administration of penicillin', *Lancet*, **i**, 387, 1943
42 Foerster, 'Sepsis im Anschluss an ausgedehnte Periporitis Heilung durch Streptozon', *Zent. Haut u. GeschlKr.*, **45**, 549, 1933
43 Foster, W. D., 'Medical History I, Sir Alexander Fleming as a bacteriologist', *Makerere Med. Jour.*, **8**, 11, 1965
44 Fuller, A., 'Is p-aminobenzene sulphonamide the active agent in Prontosil therapy?', *Lancet*, **i**, 194, 1937
45 Grutz, O., 'Beitrag zur Kenntnis der infektiös-toxischen Erythema – exsudativum multiforme – ännlichen Exanthema', *Med. Klin.*, **30**, 52, 1934
46 Hamid Ali Kahn, 'Population explosion—a paediatric problem', *Brit. Med. Jour.*, **ii**, 1475, 1966
47 Hare, R., 'Sources of haemolytic streptococcal infections of wounds in war and civil life', *Lancet*, **i**, 109, 1940
48 Hare, R., 'Almroth Edward Wright', *St Mary's Hosp. Gaz.*, **42**, 4, 1962
49 Hare, R., McClelland, L. & Morgan, J., 'A method for the concentration of influenza virus', *Can. Pub. Health Jour.*, **33**, 325, 1942
50 Hare, R. & Willits, R. E., 'The source and prevention of septic infection of wounds', *Can. Med. Assoc. Jour.*, **44**, 230, 1941
51 Hobby, G. L., Meyer, K. & Chaffee, E., 'Observations on the mechanism of action of penicillin', *Proc. Soc. Exper. Biol. Med.*, **50**, 281, 1942
52 Hoerlein, H., 'The chemotherapy of infectious diseases caused by protozoa and bacteria', *Proc. Roy. Soc. Med.*, **29**, 313, 1935–6
53 Hoerlein, H., 'The development of chemotherapy for bacterial diseases', *Practitioner*, **139**, 635, 1937
54 Jennings, M. A., *see* Florey *et al.*, 1949, p. 1152.
55 Klee, P. & Römer, H., 'Prontosil bei streptokokken Erkrankungen', *Deut. Med. Woch.*, **61**, 253, 1935
56 La Touche, C. J., Private communication
57 Lancefield, R. C. & Hare, R., 'The serological differentiation of pathogenic and non-pathogenic strains of haemolytic streptococci from parturient women', *J. Exper. Med.*, **61**, 335, 1935
58 Levaditi, C. & Vaisman, A., 'Action curative et preventive du chlorohydrate du 4'sulphamido-2,4-diamino-azobenzène dans l'infection streptococcique experimentale', *Compt. Rend. Acad. Sci.*, **200**, 1694, 1935

59 Lovell, R., Private communication
60 Masters, D., *Miracle drug*, London, Eyre & Spottiswood, 1946
61 McKinnon, N. E., Ross, M. A. & Defries, R. D., 'Reduction in diphtheria in 36,000 Toronto school children as a result of an immunization campaign', *Can. Pub. Health Jour.*, **22,** 217, 1931
62 McClelland, L. & Hare, R., 'The adsorption of influenza virus by red cells and a new in vitro method for measuring antibodies for influenza virus', *Can. Pub. Health Jour.*, **30,** 530, 1941
63 Maurois, A., *The Life of Sir Alexander Fleming*, Trans. Gerard Hopkins, London, Jonathan Cape, 1959
64 Northey, E. H., 'The sulphonamides and allied compounds', American Chemical Society Monograph No. 106, 1948
65 Parish, H. J., *A History of Immunization*, Edinburgh and London, Livingstone, 1965
66 Park, W. H., Schroder, M. C. & Zingher, A., 'The control of diphtheria', *Amer. J. Pub. Health*, **13,** 23, 1928
67 Pryce, D. M., Private communication
68 Ramon, G., 'Un siècle et demi de lutte contre la diphtérie', *Biol. Med. Paris*, **49,** 1, 1960
69 Reid, R., 'Some properties of a bacterial inhibitory substance produced by a mould', *J. Bact.*, **29,** 215, 1935
70 Ridley, F., Private communication
71 Rogers, K. B., Private communication
72 Schreus, H. Th., 'Chemotherapie des Erysipels und anderer Infektionen mit Prontosil', *Deut. Med. Woch.*, **61,** 255, 1935
73 Smith, J., 'Causation and source of infection in puerperal fever', Edinburgh, Dept. of Health for Scotland, 1931
74 Tréfouël, J., Tréfouël, J., Nitti, F. & Bovet, D., 'Activité du p-aminophénylsulfamide sur les infections expérimentales de la souris et du lapin', *Compt. Rend. Soc. Biol.*, **120,** 756, 1935
75 Wright, A. E., *A Short Treatise on Anti-Typhoid Inoculation*, Westminster, Archibald Constable, 1904
76 Wright, A. E., *Technique of the Teat and Capillary Glass Tube*, London, Constable, 1912
77 Wright, A. E., 'A lecture on the treatment of war wounds', *Lancet*, **i,** 939, 1917
78 Wright, A. E., Colebrook, L. & Storer, E. J., 'New principles in therapeutic inoculation', *Lancet*, **i,** 365, 417 and 473, 1923

Index

INDEX

GEORGE ALLEN & UNWIN LTD

Head office:
40 Museum Street, London, W.C.1
Telephone: 01-405 8577

Sales, Distribution and Accounts Departments
Park Lane, Hemel Hempstead, Herts.
Telephone: 0442 3244

Athens: 7 Stadiou Street, Athens 125
Auckland: P.O. Box 36013, Northcote Central, N.4
Barbados: P.O. Box 222, Bridgetown
Beirut: Deeb Building, Jeanne d'Arc Street
Bombay: 103/5 Fort Street, Bombay 1
Calcutta: 285J Bepin Behari Ganguli Street, Calcutta 12
Cape Town: 68 Shortmarket Street
Dacca: Alico Building, 18 Motijheel, Dacca 2
Delhi: 1/18D Asaf Ali Road, New Delhi 1
Hong Kong: 105 Wing on Mansion, 26 Hankow Road, Kowloon
Ibadan: P.O. Box 62
Karachi: Karachi Chambers, McLeod Road
Lahore: 22 Falettis' Hotel, Egerston Road
Madras: 2/18 Mount Road, Madras 2
Manila: P.O. Box 157, Quezon City D-505
Mexico: Villalongin 32, Mexico 5, D.F.
Nairobi: P.O. Box 30583
Rio de Janeiro: Caixa Postal 2537-Zc-00
Singapore: 36c Prinsep Street, Singapore 7
Sydney, N.S.W.: Bradbury House, 55 York Street
Tokyo: C.P.O. Box 1728, Tokyo 100-91
Toronto: 145 Adelaide Street West, Toronto 1

ANTHONY SMITH

The Body

Nothing quite like this book has been written before. It explores the human body, its properties, abilities, deficiencies and peculiarities in terms that the general reader can understand and the expert reader will approve.

It is not concerned with illness or dominated by medicine, but is written in a biological context, relating the human being to its evolutionary past.

It is compulsively readable, wonderfully entertaining in its numerous digressions, immensely informed, entirely up-to-date, and often drily humorous in a sophisticated and purposeful fashion. Out-of-the-way information of direct relevance pours out of every section. It describes the mechanism of the body without fear, reverence, or a pretence that mankind is all-knowing about itself. Some of the body's functions are inefficient, many aspects are unknown, but all are of intense interest to mankind.

Sex and reproduction are a central topic, because they dominate the cycle of life itself. The first half of the book traces the development of the body from conception, through pregnancy, birth and puberty to old age and death. And there are innumerable fascinating by-ways along the route. Whole sections on circumcision and suicide, blood-groups and twinning and a thousand topics of perennial interest which are seldom explored or explained. The incidence of colour blindness, the progress of haemophilia through Queen Victoria's family, the weight of a three-month-old foetus, the history of forceps and the price of human milk.

The chapters that follow are concerned with particular aspects of bodily function—the brain, sleep, speech, the five senses, the digestive system, excretion, respiration, the heart and the blood, the skeleton and its muscles. Finally, the sinister effect of radiation on the human body is explored.

Once again the evolutionary approach and an unquenchable curiosity combine to produce a unique store-house of reliable facts and lucid exposition. In conception and method Anthony Smith does for the human body what John Gunther has done for the continents of the world.

No adult man or woman could find it dull or fail to be informed by it.

'A valuable encyclopaedia of scientific knowledge. . . . It should be widely read.'

Sir Julian Huxley

'With the skill of an outstanding science writer he reveals in depth and in detail an immense amount of information and insight with a liveliness which makes it exciting reading.'

Ritchie Calder

ISAAC ASIMOV

Photosynthesis

In his customary lucid and engaging style, Isaac Asimov provides a look through the chemist's eyes at the process upon which life in all its forms is utterly dependent.

Why is it that the earth's food supply doesn't run out? What is responsible for the replenishment of the atmosphere's store of oxygen? How is sunlight transformed into usable energy?

In exploring these and other questions, Dr. Asimov clearly explains the vital process of photosynthesis and traces the efforts of scientists to understand its role in the fundamental chemistry of life.

One of the most enthusiastic expositors of science in our time, as well as an accomplished science fiction writer, Isaac Asimov is the author of numerous other works, including his *Biographical Encyclopaedia of Science and Technology* and *Understanding Physics*. He is currently Associate Professor of Biochemistry at Boston University School of Medicine.

KENNETH LANE

The Longest Art

The future success of the Health Service depends on first-class general practice and this depends on the number and quality of the young doctors who make it their career. It is therefore of great importance that the life and work of the general practitioner should be seen as it really is—as the most demanding and the most rewarding career in medicine.

Kenneth Lane's own experiences form the basis of his description of the Family Doctor's daily work, his planning, his responsibilities and above all the relationships between doctor and families.

In this personalised account he shows that the art of healing survives in the scientific age and that as long as healing depends on understanding the emotions and relationships of men and women it will remain an art.

'This is a fascinating book. What gives the book its vitality are the case histories. . . . It epitomizes the life of a family doctor.'

British Medical Journal